Rev. William C. Gaventa, MDiv
David L. Coulter, MD
Editors

End-of-Life Care:
Bridging Disability and Aging with Person-Centered Care

End-of-Life Care: Bridging Disability and Aging with Person-Centered Care has been co-published simultaneously as *Journal of Religion, Disability & Health*, Volume 9, Numbers 2 2005.

Pre-publication REVIEWS, COMMENTARIES, EVALUATIONS . . .

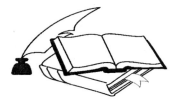

"This book simply NEEDS TO BE READ BY ALL WHO WORK WITH THE DYING OR DISABLED. . . . A valued addition to the literature in both thanatology (the study of dying) and the study of persons with disabilities. Gaventa and Coulter not only offer a sensitive analysis of the difficulties of providing good end-of-life care to persons with disabilities, they offer a paradigm that allows for compassionate and humane care."

Kenneth J. Doka, PhD
Professor of Gerontology
The College of New Rochelle
Senior Consultant
The Hospice Foundation of America

More Pre-publication
REVIEWS, COMMENTARIES, EVALUATIONS . . .

"**A**N EXTREMELY VALUABLE RESOURCE. . . . Discusses the universal and very complex question of how to achieve a good death, taking into account the unique considerations presented by disability: How do we think about disability, both consciously and subconsciously, and how do these constructs impact the end-of-life decisions we make? How can we reflect on our own lives and values in a way that can help us determine how to treat or intervene with those who have disabilities? And how do we balance the rights of those with disabilities with what *we* feel is right? This book discusses disability and the decision-making process at the end of life from philosophical, legal, psychosocial, ethical, religious, and cultural perspectives."

Dena Schulman-Green, PhD
Associate Research Scientist
Yale University School of Nursing

"**I** found this text both ENLIGHTENING AND DISTURBING. Mulitple issues are addressed. . . . Readers will be challenged to integrate ideas and concepts from special education, rehabilitation, theology, aging, social policy, law, and ethics–and to apply them not only within the mental retardation and mental health systems, but also to nursing home, hospital, and community populations. Co-Editors Gaventa and Coulter, both experts themselves in the needs of individuals and their families struggling with intellectual, behavioral, and functional disabilities, have assembled a multidisciplinary team of experts to deliberate on end-of-life issues across the lifespan."

Janet B. Craig, DHA, RN
Assistant Professor
Clemson University
Chair, Upstate SC EOL
Educational Collaborative

The Haworth Pastoral Press®
An Imprint of The Haworth Press, Inc.

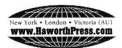

New York • London • Victoria (AU)
www.HaworthPress.com

End-of-Life Care:
Bridging Disability and Aging
with Person-Centered Care

End-of-Life Care: Bridging Disability and Aging with Person-Centered Care has been co-published simultaneously as *Journal of Religion, Disability & Health*, Volume 9, Number 2 2005.

End-of-Life Care: Bridging Disability and Aging with Person-Centered Care, edited by Rev. William C. Gaventa, MDiv, and David L. Coulter, MD (Vol. 9, No. 2, 2005). *A probing set of examinations into disability, Alzheimer's, and end-of-life debates, using a pair of cogent arguments as a starting point, followed by carefully considered responses from other experts.*

Critical Reflections on Stanley Hauerwas' Theology of Disability: Disabling Society, Enabling Theology, edited by John Swinton, PhD (Vol. 8, No. 3/4, 2004). *"AN EXCELLENT AND LONG-NEEDED RESOURCE. . . . This work will not only continue the ongoing discussion among those specializing in the theology of disability in general and disability related to intellectual development in particular, but will also serve to bring disability into the mainline of contemporary theological discussion." (Kerry H. Wynn, PhD, Director, Learning Enrichment Center, Southeast Missouri State University)*

Voices in Disability and Spirituality from the Land Down Under: From Outback to Outfront, edited by Rev. Dr. Christopher Newell, PhD, and Rev. Andy Calder (Vol. 8, No. 1/2, 2004). *"In recent years disability theology has emerged alongside Black theology and womens' theology as a new genre seeking to express the concerns of people whose experience has often been marginalized. This collection is A SIGNIFICANT AUSTRALIAN CONTRIBUTION TO THIS GROWING LITERATURE. The early explorers named Australia 'the south land of the Holy Spirit.' John M. Hull, PhD, Hon DTheol, Professor Emeritus of Religious Education, University of Birmingham, England; Author of* On Sight and Insight *and* In the Beginning There was Darkness).

Graduate Theological Education and the Human Experience of Disability, edited by Robert C. Anderson (Vol. 7, No. 3, 2003). *"A comprehensive overview of theological education and disability. . . . Concise and well written. . . . Offers rich theological insights and abundant practical advice. I strongly recommend this volume as a key introduction to this important emerging topic in theological education." (Rev. John W. Crossin, PhD, OSFS, Executive Director, Washington Theological Consortium)*

The Pastoral Voice of Robert Perske, edited by William C. Gaventa, Jr., MDiv, and David L. Coulter, MD (Vol. 7, No. 1/2, 2003). *"Must reading for seminary students and clinincal program directors. Pastors, providers, and parents concerned with persons suffering from cognitive, intellectual, and developmental disabilities will find these vigorous testimonies readable, timely, fresh, and inspiring despite having been written more than 30 years ago." (Barbara J. Lampe, JD, Executive Director, National Apostolate for Inclusion Ministry)*

Spirituality and Intellectual Disability: International Perspectives on the Effect of Culture and Religion on Healing Body, Mind, and Soul, edited by William C. Gaventa, Jr., MDiv, and David L. Coulter, MD (Vol. 5, No. 2/3, 2001). *"Must reading . . . perspectives from many faiths and cultures on the spiritual needs and gifts of people with mental retardation." (Ginny Thornburgh, EdM, Religion and Disability Program, National Organization on Disability, Washington, DC)*

The Theological Voice of Wolf Wolfensberger, edited by William C. Gaventa, MDiv, and David L. Coulter, MD (Vol. 4, No. 2/3, 2001). *This thought-provoking volume presents Wolfensberger's challenging, outrageous, and inspiring ideas on the theological significance of disabilities, including the problem with wheelchair access ramps in churches, the meaning of suffering, and the spiritual gifts of the mentally retarded.*

End-of-Life Care: Bridging Disability and Aging with Person-Centered Care

Rev. William C. Gaventa, MDiv
David L. Coulter, MD
Editors

End-of-Life Care: Bridging Disability and Aging with Person-Centered Care has been co-published simultaneously as *Journal of Religion, Disability & Health*, Volume 9, Number 2 2005.

The Haworth Pastoral Press®
An Imprint of The Haworth Press, Inc.

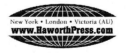

New York • London • Victoria (AU)
www.HaworthPress.com

Published by

The Haworth Pastoral Press, 10 Alice Street, Binghamton, NY 13904-1580 USA

The Haworth Pastoral Press is an imprint of The Haworth Press, Inc., 10 Alice Street, Binghamton, NY 13904-1580 USA.

End-of-Life Care: Bridging Disability and Aging with Person-Centered Care has been co-published simultaneously as *Journal of Religion, Disability & Health*, Volume 9, Number 2 2005.

The development, preparation, and publication of this work has been undertaken with great care. However, the publisher, employees, editors, and agents of The Haworth Press and all imprints of The Haworth Press, Inc., including The Haworth Medical Press® and The Pharmaceutical Products Press®, are not responsible for any errors contained herein or for consequences that may ensue from use of materials or information contained in this work. Opinions expressed by the author(s) are not necessarily those of The Haworth Press, Inc.

Cover design by Kerry E. Mack

Library of Congress Cataloging-in-Publication Data

End-of-life care: bridging disability and aging with person-centered care / William C. Gaventa, David L. Coulter, editors.
    p. cm.
"Co-published simultaneously as Journal of religion, disability & health, volume 9, number 2 2005"–T.p. verso.
    Includes bibliographical references and index.
    ISBN 13: 978-0-7890-3072 -6 (hard cover : alk. paper)
    ISBN 10: 0-7890-3072 -1 (hard cover : alk. paper)
    ISBN 13: 978-0-7890-3073 -3 (soft cover : alk. paper)
    ISBN 10: 0-7890-3073 -X (soft cover : alk. paper)
    1. Terminal care–Moral and ethical aspects. 2. Palliative treatment–Moral and ethical aspects. 3. Medicine–Decision making–Moral and ethical aspects. 4. People with mental disabilities–Medical care–Moral and ethical aspects. 5. People with mental disabilities–Legal status, laws, etc. 6. Medical ethics. I. Gaventa, William C. II. Coulter, David L. III. Journal of religion, disability & health.
R726.E485 2005
179.7–dc22   2005011857

Indexing, Abstracting & Website/Internet Coverage

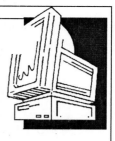

This section provides you with a list of major indexing & abstracting services and other tools for bibliographic access. That is to say, each service began covering this periodical during the year noted in the right column. Most Websites which are listed below have indicated that they will either post, disseminate, compile, archive, cite or alert their own Website users with research-based content from this work. (This list is as current as the copyright date of this publication.)

Abstracting, Website/Indexing Coverage . . . . Year When Coverage Began

- *Applied Social Sciences Index & Abstracts (ASSIA)*
  (Online: ASSI via Data-Star) (CDRom: ASSIA Plus)
  <http://www.csa.com> . . . . *
- *AURSI African Urban & Regional Science Index. A scholarly &*
  research index which synthesises & compiles all publications
  on urbanization & regional science in Africa within the world.
  Published annually 2004
- *CINAHL (Cumulative Index to Nursing & Allied Health*
  Literature), in print, EBSCO, and SilverPlatter, DataStar,
  and PaperChase (Support materials include Subject Heading List,
  Database Search Guide, and instructional video)
  <http://www.cinahl.com> 1999
- *e-psyche, LLC <http://www.e-psyche.net>* . . . . *
- *EBSCOhost Electronic Journals Service (EJS)*
  <http://ejournals.ebsco.com> 2001
- *Educational Research Abstracts (ERA) (online database)*
  <http://www.tandf.co.uk/era> 2003
- *Family & Society Studies Worldwide*
  <http://www.nisc.com> 1996
- *Family Index Database <http://www.familyscholar.com>* 2003
- *Google <http://www.google.com>* 2004
- *Google Scholar <http://scholar.google.com>* 2004
- *Haworth Document Delivery Center*
  <http://www.HaworthPress.com/journals/dds.asp> 1999
- *Human Resources Abstracts (HRA)* . . . . *

(continued)

Special Bibliographic Notes related to special journal issues (separates) and indexing/abstracting:

- indexing/abstracting services in this list will also cover material in any "separate" that is co-published simultaneously with Haworth's special thematic journal issue or DocuSerial. Indexing/abstracting usually covers material at the article/chapter level.
- monographic co-editions are intended for either non-subscribers or libraries which intend to purchase a second copy for their circulating collections.
- monographic co-editions are reported to all jobbers/wholesalers/approval plans. The source journal is listed as the "series" to assist the prevention of duplicate purchasing in the same manner utilized for books-in-series.
- to facilitate user/access services all indexing/abstracting services are encouraged to utilize the co-indexing entry note indicated at the bottom of the first page of each article/chapter/contribution.
- this is intended to assist a library user of any reference tool (whether print, electronic, online, or CD-ROM) to locate the monographic version if the library has purchased this version but not a subscription to the source journal.
- individual articles/chapters in any Haworth publication are also available through the Haworth Document Delivery Service (HDDS).

End-of-Life Care:
Bridging Disability and Aging
with Person-Centered Care

CONTENTS

ABOUT THE EDITORS

Rev. William C. Gaventa, MDiv, is Associate Professor, Department of Pediatrics, Robert Wood Johnson Medical School, and Coordinator of Community and Congregational Supports at the Elizabeth M. Boggs Center on Developmental Disabilities, the University Center of Excelence in Developmental Disabilities of New Jersey. He also coordinates a training and technical assistance team for the New Jersey Self Determination Initiative, which now supports more than 300 individuals and their families. Mr. Gaventa also served as Coordinator of Family Support for the Georgia Developmental Disabilities Council, Chaplain and Coordinator of Religious Services for the Monroe Developmental Center, and Executive Secretary for the Religion Division of the AAMR since 1985. He is serving on the Board of Directors of the AAMR, 2002-2005.

David L. Coulter, MD, is a member of the faculty of the Departments of Neurology and Social Medicine at Harvard Medical School and is afiliated with the Institute for Community Inclusion at Children's Hospital Boston. During a fellowship in ethics at Harvard Medical School, he worked to develop a broad-based spiritual basis for bioethics. When he was at the Boston Medical Center, Dr. Coulter founded a group that explored the role of spirituality in pediatrics. His research focuses on issues faced by children with disabilities and their families who belong to various cultures. Dr. Coulter was Vice-President of the American Association on Mental Retardation (AAMR) in 2002, President-Elect of AAMR in 2003, and President of AAMR in 2004.

Preface:
End of Life, Religion,
Disability, and Health:
Where All the Paths Converge

This publication is based on the premise that issues faced by people with disabilities and their families, friends, and supporters frequently raise stark and key issues that bridge the perspectives of religion/spirituality on the one hand and health care on the other. Or, in other words, disability often becomes the place where inherent, ever present, and universal questions about life, faith, and caregiving become starkly evident. That intersection is nowhere more obvious than where the various paths and perspectives from different disabilities and disciplines converge at the end of life.

Several issues ago, we published Russ Cooper-Dowda's moving account of her own journey and that of Terry Schiavo, just as Terry Schiavo was becoming a household name. In the last few months, newspapers have carried the issues around her story and the stories of euthanasia for certain kinds of children in hospitals in the Netherlands and other places. Email listservs have almost come to blows with debates about the Oscar awards going to *Million Dollar Baby* and *The Sea Inside*. The "usual suspects" in various political debates around issues with people with disabilities often end up on very different sides, or aligned with political bedfellows that seem very strange.

What's going on? Huge issues, for one, because that intersection highlights one of the dangers that many people with disabilities face, i.e., that of serving as the "canary birds in the mines" where dangerous and risky issues that impact everyone first get raised, or tested, around

[Haworth co-indexing entry note]: "Preface: End of Life, Religion, Disability, and Health: Where All the Paths Converge." Gaventa, William C., and David L. Coulter. Co-published simultaneously in Journal of Religion, Disability & Health (The Haworth Pastoral Press, an imprint of The Haworth Press, Inc.) Vol. 9, No. 2, 2005, pp. xix-xxiii; and: *End-of-Life Care: Bridging Disability and Aging with Person-Centered Care* (ed: Rev. William Gaventa, and David Coulter) The Haworth Pastoral Press, an imprint of The Haworth Press, Inc., 2005, pp. xiii-xvii. Single or multiple copies of this article are available for a fee from The Haworth Document Delivery Service [1-800-HAWORTH, 9:00 a.m. - 5:00 p.m. (EST). E-mail address: docdelivery@haworthpress.com].

Available online at http://www.haworthpress.com/web/JRDH
　　xiii

people whose quality of life is assumed to be different. Are we seeing, as Hans Reinders (2000) notes in his book, *The Future of the Disabled in Liberal Society*, a time when the inherent value assumptions of reason, freedom, and choice in a generally liberal society end up endangering the very people they also supposedly respect and protect? James Mostrom, a doctor, writing in a Syracuse paper, notes how the arguments had gotten framed as a right to die issue, when in fact the real issue is about the right of people with disabilities to live (Mostrom, 2005).

We also often hear that policy and practice issues could bridge the fields of disability and aging, but issues of stigma and value assumptions also get in the way, e.g., "I may be getting old, but at least I am not disabled." But as we move towards end-of-life issues and concerns, the "differences" fade away, and the common themes and questions emerge. How do we honor life? Caregivers? Family and friends? Related, do we even do a good job of recognizing how people with intellectual disabilities think about death, how they grieve, and those around them? How do we help individuals (with or without intellectual disabilities) prepare for their own death? How do we help those around them deal with grief and loss?

We are honored to use this volume to explore some of the questions and the dialogue. We had started to plan a collection focusing on end-of-life issues, thinking we would have to go and solicit the papers and perspectives. We were mistaken. They literally came to us, perhaps a metaphor for what will happen to all of us around these issues in one way or another.

In the summer of 2004, one of us (Bill Gaventa) had the good fortune of going to the IASSID Conference in Montpelier, where there were more than ten sessions with two or three papers or presentations in each session dealing with issues of death and grieving with people with intellectual disabilities. Rud Turnbull, Co-Director of The Beach Center, then sent us a draft of a presentation he had been asked to make as a parent, lawyer, and policy expert to the National Association of Protection and Advocacy Systems. Mary Jane Iozzio then sent a paper, from her perspective as daughter and theologian, about the caregiving issues raised for her mother and family around their care for her father with Alzheimer's. When we asked others to review their papers, their reviews, such as Stan Hauerwas', turned out to be so interesting that we decided to revise and include them in the volume so that others could be part of this dialogue. Hans Reinders just happened to be here in New Jersey for six months at the Center for Theological Inquiry. Ginny Pugh directs

Black Mountain Center, where they support both people with multiple disabilities and people with Alzheimer's.

At The Boggs Center, we were doing some work with Leigh Ann Kingsbury in Essential Lifestyle Planning when she told us how she was working on using that process in a project for end-of-life planning for people with developmental disabilities. Then the Boggs Center invited Angela King, director of the Last Passages Project, to New Jersey for one of our Developmental Disability Lecture Series. As I said, the possibilities and resources just kept coming.

David Wetherow had shared a very moving account of the final hours of life of David and Faye's daughter, Amber, on a national listserv. Then, Richard Rienstra sent me, just for my interest, Susan Harrison Wolffis' story about the funeral of his friend, Paul Novoselick. Personal experiences, conceptual theology and policy, suggested practices, responses and dialogue: the first of what may be several volumes was born. Another volume is being compiled by guest editors from the sessions on death and dying, grief, and people with intellectual disabilities from the IASSID Conference. We believe and hope that these collections will be provocative food for both our professional and personal souls.

What else will guide our thinking and prayerful/ethical action in this area with so many issues and questions? Just as this publication goes to press, David Coulter led a presentation at a conference in Atlanta, and outlined four principles from his work as a neurologist. To summarize them:

1. *All persons with I/DD (Intellectual/developmental disabilities) are valuable and deserve respect.*

Individuals with developmental disabilities do not experience their disability as a loss. People who acquire a disability (such as in a car accident) do experience a loss, but that is different. Thus persons with DD are not "suffering" from their disability. We must not project our own fears of loss onto people who have never had such a loss and conclude that their life is not worthwhile just because we would not want to live like that.

2. *We should try to find out what the person with I/DD wants (as much as possible) and honor that.*

This relates to the principle of autonomy and self-determination, of course. In biothethics, informed consent to treatment (or withdrawal of treatment) is based on three elements:

A. Information–having sufficient information upon which to make a decision.

B. Capacity–having the ability to assess the information adequately.

C. Voluntariness–being free from undue influence by others.

Thus, the challenge is to determine the authentic voice of persons with I/DD, understand the choices they have made and are making (which our field knows how to do), and place this in context.

3. *We should always act to promote the best interests of the person with I/DD.*

This relates to the ethical principle of beneficence. I talked about the need for a subjective perspective on quality of life (see the books on this topic edited by Bob Schalock) and seeing things from the point of view of the person with I/DD. I also mentioned the principle of double effect, which allows one to provide a well-intentioned treatment such as pain relief, knowing that it may have other effects that could be life-limiting.

From a spiritual perspective, I also mentioned that continued life is not always the highest good. For a Christian, salvation is the highest good, and reconciliation with God may be more important than continued life. The best interest of a Christian with I/DD may well be the assurance of a personal relationship with God and "saving one's soul."

4. *Physicians should not kill.*

This relates to the ethical principle of non-maleficence. The question here is what are the allowable options at the end of life. The focus should be on palliative care and hospice (true "caring at the end of life") rather than termination of life. "Rational suicide" is probably permissible (as in the movie MDB), but physician-assisted suicide is not. Withdrawal of life-sustaining treatment such as nutrition and hydration may be permissible in highly selected situations (primarily true PVS) but not in other states of limited consciousness (as in Terry Schiavo's case). Euthanasia is never permissible, particularly when decided by surrogates (such as parents asking to have their child's life terminated).

Where do we hope this discussion goes? For one, David Coulter will be working with others to develop a policy statement for the AAMR and other organizations related to end-of-life care. See for yourself the policy recommendations from the Last Passages Project, which they have graciously allowed us to reprint in this issue, along with their resource list. As you read this collection, let your reflections and thinking be guided by your relationships with others, as each author in this volume has labored to integrate their personal experience with their professional expertise. "How do we integrate love and public policy?", as my boss Deborah Spitalnik at The Boggs Center provocatively asked last spring in an address for our 20th Anniversary. It is not easy work, as Hans Reinders so pointedly says in his response to Rud Turnbull, because most of us are not at all certain about what we want and think about our own end-of-life questions, much less those for the people whom we love and support.

William C. Gaventa, MDiv
David L. Coulter, MD
Co-Editors

REFERENCES

Mostrom, J. (2005). Solitary confinement: Why you and I should care about Terri Schiavo. Syracuse: Post Standard, Opinion Page. For the full Letter to the Editor, go to: *http://www.syracuse.com/opinion/poststandard/index.ssf?/base/opinion-5/110 9669932182430.xml*

Reinders, H. (2000). *The future of the disabled in liberal society*. South Bend: University of Notre Dame Press.

What Should We Do for Jay?
The Edges of Life and Cognitive Disability

H. Rutherford Turnbull III, JD

SUMMARY. This article asks who, how, and on what grounds end-of-life decisions should be made for a person with a significant cognitive disability (the author's son). It argues that the decisions must be based on principled grounds and that those grounds are both legal (the core concepts of disability policy and the appropriate case law). It describes how five different "models" of thinking about disability affect our decision-making, and how those models reflect as much about the decision-makers as about people with disabilities. It next poses the paradox that we may make the right decision for the wrong reason, or the wrong decision for the right reason. Finally, it argues that we should yield to the paradoxes, affirm but move beyond rights, and embrace trust and compassion as supplementary grounds for decision-making. *[Article copies available for a fee from The Haworth Document Delivery Service: 1-800-HAWORTH. E-mail address: <docdelivery@haworthpress.com> Website: <http://www.HaworthPress.com> © 2005 by The Haworth Press, Inc. All rights reserved.]*

KEYWORDS. End-of-life, intellectual disability, disability policy, family and friends, compassion and trust

---

H. Rutherford Turnbull III is Co-Founder and Co-Director, Beach Center on Disability, The University of Kansas, Lawrence, KS 66045.
Printed with permission.

[Haworth co-indexing entry note]: "What Should We Do for Jay? The Edges of Life and Cognitive Disability." Turnbull, H. Rutherford. Co-published simultaneously in Journal of Religion, Disability & Health (The Haworth Pastoral Press, an imprint of The Haworth Press, Inc.) Vol. 9, No. 2, 2005, pp. 1-25; and: *End-of-Life Care: Bridging Disability and Aging with Person-Centered Care* (ed: Rev. William C. Gaventa, and David L. Coulter) The Haworth Pastoral Press, an imprint of The Haworth Press, Inc., 2005, pp. 1-25. Single or multiple copies of this article are available for a fee from The Haworth Document Delivery Service [1-800-HAWORTH, 9:00 a.m. - 5:00 p.m. (EST). E-mail address: docdelivery@haworthpress.com].

Available online at http://www.haworthpress.com/web/JRDH
doi:10.1300/J095v9n02_01

INTRODUCTION

Jay Turnbull, my son, is a 37-year-old man with low-moderate mental retardation, rapid cycling bi-polar disability, mild autism, and a chronic heart ailment. He has no legal guardian. Accordingly, Ann and I, as his natural guardians, have been acting as his surrogates, with his assent, for the entire period of his adulthood. We have been using a series of private contracts between us (as his surrogates) and his health-care and commercial providers. Under these contracts, his providers agree with us that we may act on Jay's behalf and for his benefit, the providers will secure his consent to the treatment he needs, to the maximum extent they are able to do so, with our assistance, and the providers thereby contract with us, not Jay, to treat him. He is the third-party beneficiary of a contract and the direct beneficiary of the services.

The contract exists by reason of the fact that Jay, Ann, and I are under the care of the same internal-medicine physician, dentist, and surgeon. These professionals not only know us and our relationship with and commitment to Jay, but they also trust us to act in Jay's best interests, not our own. Moreover, we have always been consulted by Jay's psychiatrist about Jay's treatment, and this physician also approaches his treatment for Jay with the same reliance on us as Jay's (and our) other providers do. Each of these three providers make every effort to secure Jay's consent, and they usually succeed. Jay says "yes" and physically consents to their treatment, but it is arguable that he fully understands the nature of their treatment, especially when it involves psychotropic medication.

It is clear that neither Ann nor I will outlive Jay. He is 30 years younger than I and 20 years younger than Ann. So we must project a situation in which the decision is stark and simple: how to accede to his needs and wishes when he is at the end of his life? Who will decide what to do, by what standards will they decide, and under what procedures?

Let us assume the following, rather typical, scenario. A competent and caring physician has certified that Jay is within six months of death. The physician's judgment is indisputable. There is no reasonable probability of reversing the course of any condition that will end Jay's life. He has not been declared "brain dead" or "organ dead." He is not in state custody. Someone other than Ann and I, or one of us, must make a decision concerning what to do for him during the rest of his life and what, if any, medical treatment or other interventions, such as Hospice Care, will be provided or not provided to him.

We must also assume that his sisters, Amy and Kate, and his personal care attendants, Bryan and Tom, will be involved in the decision-making, as will his close friends in our small community and his physician. If they have paid close attention to my thinking about these matters, they will be guided by a decision-making framework that my colleague Matt Stowe and I developed. In that framework, we identified the core concepts of disability policy and the overarching principles that organize those core concepts (Turnbull & Stowe, 2001).

They must also bear in mind Jay's cognitive disability. The fact that he has a disability is a distinction that makes a difference in how any of us deal with each other; the fact that he has a cognitive disability is itself a particular distinction that makes a particular distinction. It requires special care and scrutiny: the greater the cognitive disability and the greater the risk, intrusiveness, and irreversibility of a decision, the more the decision requires scrutiny to know whether it adheres to the core concepts and overarching principles of disability policy (Turnbull, 1978). So, what shall we do for Jay?

In this article, I set out, first, the guiding principles and, second, the case law related to them. By placing the principles and cases into the context of cognitive disability and family-friend relationships, I address the issues that are peculiar to families of people with cognitive disabilities and I call special attention to how many families, ours included, make decisions for all of our "Jays." I then describe five models that inform our views of the construct we call "disability" and how these models affect our decision-making. I argue that the principles, cases, family issues, and models require us to reflect on ourselves and our relationships to disability and to our family who have disabilities.

Next, I suggest a paradox: we may make the right decision for the wrong reason, or the wrong decision for the right reason. Finally, recognizing how insufficient our principles, cases, and models can be, and how painful the paradoxes can be, I ask us not to abandon our principles and models. Instead, I ask us to retain them and to yield to the paradoxes by moving beyond rights to two elements that powerfully shape our relationships with our family and others–trust and compassion.

I do not propose to give answers, but, more, to perturb us and impel us to think hard about the hardest part of our relationships with our family, namely, the permanency of death. I urge us to think deeply about the warrants, or justifications, that our lives and our relationships with each other give for the end-of-life decisions that someone other than Ann and I must make for Jay.

I do not address the situation in which the person with a cognitive disability lacks any family members or has been abandoned by his family members. Some of the principles I discuss, however, may assist those who are charged with making decisions for those individuals.

THE GUIDING PRINCIPLES

The first question for these decision-makers is this: What standards, criteria, or principles guide them in making a decision? There are several groups of principles, at least as my colleagues and I see it (Turnbull & Stowe, 2001; Umbarger, Stowe, & Turnbull, 2004; Stowe, Turnbull, & Umbarger, 2004).

Medical Principles. Jay's physicians will argue that there are three over-riding medical principles. *Beneficence* (the "good action") and non-maleficence (not taking a "bad action") direct the physicians to help Jay and not to hurt him. Should they assist in his death, and, if so, how? Will their assistance help or hurt him; will they ease his dying or make him dead? *Autonomy* consists of three elements. First, there is physicians' freedom to exercise defensible medical judgment. Second, there is their expectation that non-professionals and the courts will defer to their judgment. Third, there is their expectation that their decision will be balanced against Jay's autonomy to determine the nature and extent of the treatment his physicians may render. When the patient, Jay, has a cognitive disability, however, that autonomy must be exercised by others. Finally, *Justice* asserts that Jay, without regard to his abilities or disabilities, has a right to appropriate health-care.

Constitutional Principles. Among Jay's close friends are several lawyers. They will argue that there are three over-riding constitutional principles. *Life* includes both Jay's sanctity of life (his substantive due process claim grounded in a negative-rights theory: do not take my life without just cause) and his quality of life (a positive-rights claim: provide me with appropriate health-care, at all stages of my life, including the end-stages of my life). *Liberty* includes Jay's right to decide for himself how to live and conclude his life. The liberty principle equates with the principles of privacy (in decision-making) and autonomy (choice) and is manifest in the legal doctrine of consent. In the disability field, autonomy and consent are comparable to such constructs as choice, empowerment/participatory decision-making, and self-determination. *Equality* holds that Jay, like all people, without regard to the nature or extent of their disability, should have equal opportunities with others. The principle is expressed in terms of equal protection (a legal doctrine), egalitarianism (a political doctrine), and normalization/social role valorization (a human rights doctrine); it is manifest in anti-discrimination laws.

Ethical Principles. Also among Jay's friends are professors of philosophy and his pastors. They concur with each other that there are three over-riding ethical principles. *Dignity* compels others to treat Jay respectfully by honoring his legal and ethical claims, including his expectation that others will treat him with dignity and respect. *Family as foundation* acknowledges that for Jay, as for minors and many adults who have cognitive disabilities, his family is the core social unit in his life and the ultimate decision-maker because it has transmitted values that Jay is presumed to adopt; there is no evidence that he has lived a life that is counter to those values and that therefore his family's values should not be imputed to him. *Community* is more than just a place where Jay lives; it also is the interaction between Jay and other individuals. Community refers to Jay's physical presence among us and to the psychological dimensions of his life among us, to the empathetic reciprocity and mutual expectations of care, compassion, and dignity.

Disability Principles. Also among Jay's friends are members of various family and professional organizations in the field of mental retardation, including The Arc and AAMR. These friends may rely on the position statements of The Arc and AAMR (2002), asserting that there are seven principles.

Rights means that Jay has a right to have health care be available (which includes the concept of "timely" care), accessible (physically, linguistically, culturally, and so on), appropriate (which includes the standards of comprehensive and medically effective), affordable, and accountable (which includes the concept of meeting legal, professional/peer, and family standards of care). This principle is consistent with the principles of beneficence, non-maleficence, justice, and equality.

Disability irrelevancy holds that Jay's disability per se may not be taken into account when people make decisions for or about him; the only factors that may be taken into account are his medical condition and general welfare. This principle is also consistent with the principles of justice and equality.

Reasonable accommodations are those supports that Jay is entitled to have because he does not have the ability to make this particular health care decision; these accommodations include guardianship, surrogate decision-making, and protection and advocacy. This principle is consistent with the principles of justice, equality, and liberty/autonomy of the person.

Consent holds that decisions (whether by Jay or a surrogate) must be informed, voluntary, and derived from a person who is legally competent (the person or a surrogate). This principle is consistent with the principle of liberty/autonomy of the person.

Surrogacy, namely, surrogate decision-making, is necessary because Jay may not have been competent to make legally effective advance directives or to make certain decisions now. This principle is consistent with the principles of autonomy.

Best interests requires a surrogate to make a decision that is in Jay's "best interests"; it disallows decisions that primarily address the interests of other people or entities. This principle is consistent with the principle of beneficence, non-maleficence, and dignity.

Edges of life decisions involve the refusal of medical treatment, nutrition, or hydration; when the refusal will result in the death of the individual, the legal authority of Jay's surrogate must be limited to those situations in which his condition is terminal, death is imminent, and any continuation or provision of treatment, nutrition, or hydration would only serve to prolong his dying or cause unconscionable suffering. In those situations, Jay has a right to aggressive medical treatment to relive pain, sustenance as medically indicated, and care designed to (and effective to) relieve his isolation, fear, and physical discomfort. This principle is consistent with the principles of beneficence, non-maleficence, life, and dignity.

I feel obliged to disclose that I have been a senior officer of AAMR and The Arc, have had a role in drafting both the Principles of Treatment of Disabled Newborns (1983), which have been incorporated into the regulations implementing the federal child-protection law, Child Abuse Prevention, Adoption, and Treatment Act, and also The Arc's policy positions, which are based on those Principles; and that I have been an advocate for people with cognitive disabilities to have the benefit of the constitutional rights I have identified. Naturally, I am loathe to turn my back to any of these constitutional rights, ethical claims, or policy statements. Yet I believe that, however necessary they are for our decision-making about Jay, they are not sufficient. I also recognize that the many people who will be involved in Jay's life and end-of-life decision making will rely on various standards; fortunately these many principles are consistent with each other. These people, however, may not agree with each other, either about the principle on which they should decide or how to apply a consensus principle. So they may seek guidance from decisions that courts have reached in comparable situations. They want to act legally and defensibly in case someone challenges their decision. I find comfort in that fact.

CASE LAW

There are several precedents and underlying principles on which the decision makers may rely. The fundamental law of the country, the Constitution, requires us to consider constitutional law first.

Constitutional Law. The United States Supreme Court has refused to acknowledge that Jay or anyone else has either a constitutional autonomy right to assisted suicide or a constitutional equal protection right to be treated, in dying, as one who is able to exercise the same rights to not refuse life-prolonging treatment as one has when the issue is not dying and life-prolonging treatment (*Washington v. Glucksburg* 1997; *Vacco v. Quill,* 1997). The Court has said that these "privacy" matters are issues that state legislatures must determine.

Procedural Due Process and State Custody. The Court has held that, when a state has guardianship over an incompetent person and also has physical custody of the person, and when the person has not executed legally valid advance directives, the state may require a high degree of proof (more than the preponderance of the evidence) that Jay or any other person would have decided to refuse life-sustaining treatment (*Cruzan v. Director*, 1990). Jay may or may not be in state custody. Still, the principle seems useful: his decision-makers should have a great deal of evidence that he would not want to continue to live as he is living at the time they must make a decision for him.

Surrogate Decision Making Standards and Procedures When a Person is in State Custody. The Massachusetts Supreme Judicial Court has held that, when an individual (Jay) is incompetent to make a decision, is terminally ill, and is in state custody, the surrogate decision-makers must make the decision that the person would make if he were competent to make a decision and could take into account his own incompetence (*Superintendent v. Saikewicz*, 1977). This is a subjective standard, not an objective 'reasonable person' standard. It requires the surrogates to determine what "warrant" or "justification" Jay's life gives. They must ask (and be sure of the answer): What evidence is available in Jay's life from which the surrogates may determine what he would want and how he would decide (if able to decide).

Legal Standards and Procedures When a Person Is not in State Custody. State abuse, neglect, and maltreatment/exploitation statutes protect Jay as a person with a disability. These incorporate federal law (Child Abuse Prevention and Treatment and Adoption Act) because the state receives federal aid conditioned on agreement to abide by the federal law. The federal regulations implementing the law (50 Fed. Register 14878-14901, Apr. 15, 1985) adopt the so-called "Baby Doe" Statement of Principles of Treatment of Disabled Newborns (1983), which I helped to draft.

This principle creates a presumption in favor of treating Jay. The presumption can be rebutted in three circumstances: (1) Jay is irreversibly comatose. (2) The intervention would be painful, beyond benefit, and border on cruelty. (3) The intervention would be ineffective to prevent Jay's death. In addition, medical malpractice standards and peer-review (IRB) procedures and standards create a professional standard that constitutes a form of legal protection for him.

As is true for the constitutional and ethical principles, so also for these: I do not turn my back to them, and, more, I hope that Jay's surrogate decision-makers will apply them for his benefit should that time and circumstance arise.

APPLYING THESE PRINCIPLES

Jay's decision makers now must apply these various principles and case law to Jay at the end of his life. Here are the factors that I believe should guide them.

Personal Autonomy. Jay's autonomy warrants respect and deference. The medical principle of autonomy says so; the constitutional principle of liberty, with its subsumed principle of autonomy, says so. The decisions in *Cruzan* and *Saikewicz* interpret and apply the constitutional principle of autonomy and implement the medical principle of autonomy. As the court noted in *Saikewicz*, to deny Jay the right to choose violates his constitutional right to equal treatment under the Fourteenth Amendment. It also violates the professional principle of justice because a denial treats him as unworthy of access to services, including the refusal of services.

Matters become more complicated, however, when the decision makers take into account Jay's relationship with his family, especially his sisters, who survive Ann and me. Our family's autonomy is entitled to respect and deference, consistent with the ethical principle that

the family is the foundational social unit of society. This principle
rests on the bonds that derive from the biological bonds and psychological commitments of family members to each other. It also rests on
the fundamental liberty right of a family to make decisions about its
members *(Troxel v. Granville, 2000; Elk Grove Unified School District v. Newdow, 2004)*.

Jay has a privacy right to be left alone when not in state custody and
to decide what to do or not do with his life, so long as he does not injure
others. In every way, the principle of privacy connects to the principle
of autonomy; the two are inseparable and thus all of the principles that
buttress autonomy also buttress privacy. Moreover, Jay's privacy/au-
tonomy principles/rights implement a different constitutional principle.

That is the principle of the least drastic means (also known as the
least restrictive means or environment): when government has a legiti-
mate reason to act, it must act in the ways that are least restrictive of a
person's liberty. The decision that Jay's surrogates should make, then,
are the ones that conform to Jay's wishes (*Saikewicz*) and that are consistent with how Ann and I, and Amy and Kate, have directed others to
deal with us.

Not only does Jay have a claim to privacy and autonomy; our family
does, too. Thus, Amy and Kate have a right to decide for him, without
state interference, so long as they do not violate any of the Baby Doe
standards. Because Jay, Amy, and Kate have been raised together and
therefore share similar values, it is right and proper to rely on Amy and
Kate to decide for Jay.

Equality, Justice, Advance Directives, and Dignity. Jay has executed
several advance directives. Here, the constitutional principle of equality
applies; he should have an opportunity to execute advance directives
and his directives should be honored, just as they would be if he were a
person without a disability. By extension, the professional principle of
justice applies; it advances equal treatment for all patients. Moreover,
his advance directives signify that he has exercised his rights of autonomy (liberty and privacy). If Jay has not executed advance directives,
the question then becomes one of disability discrimination: the denial of
an equal opportunity to have access to advance directives. Because he
has not been denied the opportunity to execute advance directives, the
following questions arise.

The law presumes that an adult is competent. That presumption fa-
vors Jay and his advance directives: he is presumed competent and his
directives are presumed to be valid. Despite the presumptions, however,
it is not certain that his health-care providers and the state (if Jay is in

state custody) will honor Jay's directives. They will ask: Was Jay really competent to execute the directives? So the question is whether the directives are really enforceable: will the physicians honor them and will the courts enforce them?

I hope that presumption in favor of the instruments' validity will govern, or if not govern then certainly guide, his surrogate decision makers. Jay knows what he wants; he may not be fully able to express it, but he knows and is entitled to his judgment about himself.

If Jay's directives are not enforceable both on the street and in the courts, then they are merely hollow symbols of Jay's autonomy, and their unenforceability, in the sense that they will not "work" for Jay, constitutes one type of disability discrimination, violates the constitutional principle of equality and of the professional principle of justice, and denies Jay the benefit of the constitutional principle of autonomy and the professional principle of justice. Arguably, these denials also violate the ethical principle of dignity. That is so because the denials disrespect the Jay's wishes, whether expressed verbally through an advance directive or expressed behaviorally through his life as he has lived it. It pains me to think of someone violating these principles when deciding about Jay.

Beneficence and Non-Maleficence; Professional Autonomy, Decision-Making, and Health-Care Decision-Makers. The principle of beneficence requires health-care providers to do good to Jay; the principle of non-maleficence requires them not to harm him. Neither principle is easy to apply. That is so because at least the following factors come into play in the decision by Jay's physicians and others to continue or discontinue treatments and other interventions. Although I recognize the power of each of these factors to influence Jay's surrogates, I also believe that beneficence requires a health-care provider to defer to Jay's autonomy (as I have laid it out above).

The Right to Treatment. Jay's right to treatment requires his physicians to treat him. Here, the imperative is not technological: it is legal. There is no right without a corresponding duty. In carrying out their duty, his physicians may use, and may argue that they must use, any technology that has been proven to be effective; indeed, they may argue that they must even use any technology that may be effective but has not yet been proven to be effective. Their first argument is based on the technology's demonstrated efficacy; their second is based on the hope that the technology will be effective, and hope leads us to other considerations.

The Prospect for Remission. Everyone may hope that, whether with or without the technology, Jay will recover and return to a status quo ante bellum (the war against disease and death).

Sanctity of Life. All may adhere to a steadfast, unshakable belief in the sanctity of life and fear that they should not play God (even though, by continuing the intervention, they do so). Here, the principle of dignity comes into play, more so than other principles such as beneficence and non-maleficence.

Quality of Life. All may recognize that Jay has lived well, that he is at the end of life, and that his life's quality is, ironically, enhanced by its termination. Again, this is a matter of dignity, but of other principles, too.

The Technological Imperative. This phrase describes the situation that physicians often face: when a technology exists, they must use it to cure disease or prevent death. Will Jay's physicians follow this imperative, and, if so, do they conform to beneficence and non-maleficence, or not? Does it depend on the technology and its efficacy to improve Jay's health and prolong his life? Probably so.

The Promethean Syndrome. This is the concept that can conquer nature and use technology to overcome that which Nature/God has willed. Here, for example, Jay's decision makers may decide to use nutrition and hydration to prolong his life (his *viva in extreme*). They already use technology to create a better body (medical rehabilitation and the bionic person–*viva in esse*) and they use human genome research to create a more perfect life/person that will exist (*viva in futuro*). Are Jay's health-care providers affected by this syndrome? If so, and if they act on it, the same questions arise here as arise with respect to the technological imperative.

The "Experimental" or "Clinical Trial" Approach. His health-providers may ask: if we use the technology, what result will we get? Here, Jay may become a "laboratory" for an "experimenter/researcher" and thus an (mere) instrument for another's benefit. Is that result beneficent? For whom?

The Fear of Malpractice. Physicians may fear that their decision will be challenged in the courts as inconsistent with professional practice and thus as malpractice and a violation of the professional principle of "non-maleficence" and the legal standard of professional care.

Evidence and Warrants for Action; Consent, Incompetence, Assent, and Multi-Lateral/Surrogate Decision-Making. If Jay was not competent at the time of executing his advance directive, the same questions and decision-making complications arise but they are compounded by other factors.

Evidence, Warrants for Action, and the Case Law. Cruzan requires the decision makers to evaluate Jay's life and to take their direction from it; his life is their warrant for acting. But it also allows a state to require the evidence to be beyond the "preponderance" level and to be clear, cogent, and convincing: more evidence than is required in a regular civil action but less than in a criminal action. So, how much evidence is necessary for Jay's decision-makers to have in order to make a decision and then to implement the decision? So long as the Jay's surrogates include his sisters and circle of friends, I will be satisfied with evidence that meets the "preponderance" test: just enough to persuade the trier of fact in a civil case. If these are the surrogates, they will not be helped, and they may indeed be hindered, by a standard of "clear, cogent, and convincing" or "beyond a reasonable doubt."

What kind of evidence suffices? In *Cruzan*, verbal statements were available. So, they must recall what Jay said and, indeed, whether he said anything at all. What if Jay was not able to make those kinds of statements? What if the only evidence is how he lived his life?

In that situation, *Saikewicz* comes into play and the decision makers must look to Jay's behavior as a form of communication and thus to behavior as a warrant for their decision-making. Jay's life in its totality is the only evidence of what he would want and how the he would decide. His behavior is communication; both oral and written communication, and behavior, provide a warrant for action. In Jay's case, who are the persons who have observed his life most closely? They are his sisters and his circle of friends. Does it matter how, how much, or how recently they have been involved in his life? Yes, but his circle is a constant circle, always involved with him; and his sisters have had at least 22 years of living with Jay on which to base their judgments.

Consent and Assent. Consent is a legal construct that advances Jay's fundamental liberty and privacy rights. When it is exercised by another person on his behalf, a legal fiction comes into play, for Jay, who (we will assume for the sake of this discussion) cannot exercise the consent, is deemed to have exercised it through the surrogate, and of course (as we assume, *arguendo*) that is a fiction, for Jay never really gave legally effective consent.

The disability rights movement has attempted to enforce Jay's consent rights and avoid surrogate decision-making by creating another legal construct, "assent." Assent is not the same as the legal concept of consent. That is so because consent requires Jay to be competent (which, *arguendo*, we assume he is not). Assent, on the other hand, involves a situation in which Jay approves the surrogate's consent, either verbally or behaviorally.

The legal concept of consent is fully legal and wholly binary: either the person has full capacity to consent or the person lacks (all or some) capacity to consent, and the contract exists between the person and a second party. By contrast, the concept of assent is a-legal and not exactly binary: it is neither legally traditional and sanctioned, nor is it traditionally illegal and prohibited, and it involves Jay, one or more other individuals acting as his natural guardians or in some other surrogate capacities, and the person who relies on Jay and his surrogates. It is a pragmatic approach to taking action in the middle ground between full competence and some degree of incompetence. Assent is almost always what Jay and his family, personal care attendants, physicians, and other care-givers use to regulate their relationships and provide benefits for Jay. Here, there are two options.

First, Jay (thus, others with cognitive disabilities) has an involved family, his family members are legally competent to consent, and Jay has almost always assented to their decisions, including such significant ones as where and how to reside and work and what kinds of medical treatment to receive or not receive. The power of Jay's family to decide derives from the ethical principle of family as foundation. (Here, we must assume that all of the closely related members of a family–spouse, domestic partner, siblings, parents, and others who have been involved regularly and significantly in Jay's life–concur with each other. When they do not, other legal issues arise, but these issues of conflict do not apply in Jay's case.)

Second, Jay (thus, too, others with cognitive disabilities) does not have family involved; instead, he has relied on other care-givers who have been part of his life and know him well. This was the *Saikewicz* situation and may well be the situation when a person has been in state custody or out of state custody but in the care (under the protection and advocacy) of other individuals, such as those who have been in Jay's circle of friends. The friends' power to decide derives from the ethical principle of community.

The ethical principle of community recognizes both the physical and the emotional/psychological bonds that develop among people. It acknowledges that people enter into "intentional communities" with each other, whether or not they share the same residence. It is analogous to the French-Spanish concept of the family council: the members of the family constitute a deliberative body that has authority to make decisions for family members who are unable to decide for themselves. It thus has some relationships to the ethical principle of family as foundation. These circles or councils occur when, for example, a person has lived in an intentional community such as a Camphill community or L'Arche community. They also occur when the person, such as Jay, has lived and worked in a community for many years, with support from house-mates (personal care attendants) and others (at work, in social/recreational activities, and in religious communities/congregations).

In these circles, councils, or communities, we impute to Jay the values of his biological family members and of the people who have been intimately involved in his life, with his family's consent. We do that because Jay has agreed to live with the support, protection, and advocacy of these circle/council members. His life among them is the evidence that *Cruzan* and *Saikewicz* require us to seek and authorize us to rely on.

Conflicts of Interest. In nearly all cases of surrogate decision making, especially at the edges of life, lies real or perceived conflicts of interest. These conflicts are based on economic, care-giving, and psychological-burden dimensions. The nature and extent of any conflict of interest are subject to scrutiny; that is so because "good" decision-making should focus on Jay, not on others, per *Saikewicz* and *Cruzan*. The only way to rule out the effect of these conflicts is to scrutinize the surrogate's decisions in order to determine whether the surrogate is making a decision that is more consistent with the person's preferences than with the surrogate's.

It is difficult to know just how much scrutiny must be brought to bear. Long ago, AAMR suggested an approach (Turnbull, 1978): as the levels of risk, irreversibility, and intrusiveness of any intervention increase and as the person's ability to consent or assent decreases, the level of scrutiny must increase. This is not inconsistent with the approach that the state (Missouri) adopted in *Cruzan* and that the Supreme Court approved: a higher level of evidence (more than preponderance) must obtain before a decision to discontinue life-maintaining intervention can be carried out. As I have noted, I prefer the ordinary "preponderance" test so long as Jay's surrogates are his family and circle of friends.

The conflicts will always exist; they do so because rarely do families and other circle members always and continuously adhere to the principle of sanctity of life, the idea that life qua life must always be preserved, whatever form the life takes and whatever the costs are to the person or others.

At some point, surrogates come to a quality of life judgment. They are permitted to do so by the *Cruzan* and *Saikewicz* cases; the constitutional principle of life (which encompasses the quality of life elements); the Baby Doe principles as adopted by AAMR (2002) and The Arc (2002) in their policy statements; the medical-professional principles of beneficence, non-maleficence, and autonomy; the ethical principles of family as foundation; the ethical principle of family as foundation (as in the *Cruzan* case, where the family sought to discontinue the life-maintaining intervention); the legal principle of equality, which prevents us from with-holding from the person the same (imputed/fictional) autonomy that competent people enjoy and exercise through advance directives; and the ethical principle of dignity, which tells some of us that death with dignity is preferable to life in insufferable and hopeless distress.

MODELS FOR DECISION-MAKING

So much of our thinking about Jay and others with disabilities derives from the "models" that we incorporate, consciously or not, about the construct called "disability" and about those affected by it. There are five different models (Turnbull & Stowe, 2001). Each points us into certain policy decisions; each may relate to Jay and the decisions we make for him at the end of his life.

Human Capacity Model. This model directs our attention to Jay's ability to acquire greater capacity and our ability to assist him to do so. The sub-models are the medical, developmental/educational, and psychological models. When we decide whether or, if so, how to intervene at the edges of Jay's life, we take into account his ability to have increased capacity and our ability to contribute to that capacity. The human capacity model underlies the presumptions in favor of treatment, education, and intervention and the *Cruzan*, *Saikewicz*, Baby Doe, and The Arc and AAMR quality of life position statements.

However much fault we may find with a theory that a person's quality of life consists of the sum of the contributions that home/family and society can make to the person, many of us (and our professional associations, such as The Arc and AAMR) come to accept a quality-of-life judgment when life is inevitably ending. The question is, always: when is that time reached? And who is to say—only his physicians, or the members of his circle/council, after consulting with trusted physicians? The time is sometime within the last six months of Jay's life, and the "who" are his sisters and his circle of friends.

The Public Law Model. This model is best reflected in edges of life decision making by the "legal rights" and "economic" sub-models, which call our attention to Jay's rights (see the Constitutional Principles) and the economic consequences to him, ourselves as individuals, and the public fisc, of any decision we make. If we decide what rights Jay has (consent, assent, treatment/intervention, refusal of treatment/intervention), we apply this model. If we consider the conflicts of interest that arise from our financial/economic relationships to Jay and the costs and benefits of various interventions, policies, and decisions, we rely on the economic sub-model.

The "Cultural" Model. This model asks us to examine the nature of our culture and whether we act consistently with it. When parents have been continuously and positively involved in our children's lives, as Ann and I have been in Jay's, we may ascribe to Jay the culture that we ourselves adopt. We also may do the same with respect to Amy and Kate. There is no evidence that they reject the cultural values that Ann and I, and Jay, adopt. Indeed, because Jay has lived consistently with that culture, we may be certain that he himself adopts it and would want decisions about the end of his life to be guided by it.

Different subcultures within our country place different values on life and dying/death. That is a complicating factor at the edges of life. One culture may "rage" against "the dying of the light "(Thomas, 1957) and do all it can to postpone the inevitable. Another may regard death as a passage, as a stage in various lives.

Another complicating factor is that cultural norms may also may be grounded in our "disability" culture, in the acknowledgement that there is a culture, a subpopulation, that consists of people with disabilities and that their collective (or purportedly representative) perspectives should control our decisions. Even within the disability subpopulation, however, there are polarized perspectives about whether medical assistance to stay alive or to die is acceptable. Some say it is; the final act of autonomy is choosing how to die, or (in Jay's case), having that choice made for us. Some say it is not; the final act of dependency is being "assisted" to die under medical supervision.

The "Technological" Model. This model asserts that a proper use of technology is to prevent or cure disability (make it disappear) and, failing that, to change the physical and other environments in which Jay and other people with disabilities live. The purpose of technology as an intervention technique, and not as a prevention technique, is to eliminate barriers to Jay's full citizenship and participation and, more, to enhance his ability to participate in the aspects of American life that he chooses to participate in. Industrial engineering and the science of ergonomics, architecture, and assistive and computer technologies are sub-models of this model. When we take into account life at the edges and the use of medical technology and the technological imperative, we work from this model. The question, though, remains: Just how much technology should we bring to bear in the final weeks of Jay's life? I think the answer lies in placing other models over the technological model. Technology is a means, not an end; it serves other values and should not drive them.

The "Theological/Ethical" Model. This model regards the construct of disability and the lives of those affected by it in either a deity-related way (our relationship to God or another deity) or in an ethically principled way (absent a theological perspective and deliberately agnostic). When we decide what "God wills" or "what is right" at the edges of life, we rely on this model. If we ask Jay where his grandparents are ("Where is Granddaddy Turnbull, Grandmother Ruth, and A-Dad Patterson?"), he will tell us, with confidence, "They are in Heaven with Baby Jesus." He has learned what we taught him, and his faith is simple and sure.

The public debate will always be about whether we, Jay's family and friends of his own faith, may make our theological or ethical choices free of public intervention and also whether, when it is Jay's life, not ours, that is the focus of our attention, we may make our decisions for him (and thus ourselves) free of public intervention. If there is a role for public intervention, the question is this: whose theology or ethic prevails if there is a conflict between our own and that of others in the public domain, such as courts, legislatures, and executives? Liberty and privacy include the right to be free of others' judgments, to exercise our own judgments, and to have Jay's judgment be exercised by us for him.

These models sometimes complement each other but they also sometimes conflict with each other. Certainly, our ways of thinking about life at the edges reflect any one or more of these models.

JAY'S LIFE AT THE EDGE
AND OUR OWN SELF-REFERENTIAL REFLECTIONS

Self-Referential Reflections. These five models do more than tell us how we think about disability as a construct, Jay, and other people with cognitive disabilities. They also reveal how we think about ourselves, our children or other "circle members" with disabilities, "disability" as a construct, the quality of life of people with disabilities before they reach the edges of life, and the edges-of-life choices that we will make for ourselves and them.

Are we more concerned, for example, with developing our maximum capacities (the human development model) than with assuring that we have certain rights (the public law model)? What has been our approach with respect to Jay? Is our decision about how to live shaped more by our families and their histories (a cultural model) than by our sense of our relationship to God (a theological model) or our sense of right/wrong (an ethical model)? What is our approach with respect to Jay? How do these models complement each other; how do they differ from and even conflict with each other; and, if they conflict, which one(s) prevail over others? Which model has prevailed over others as Jay has made his own decisions or as we have made decisions with or for him? So, as we think about Jay at the edges of his life, we invariably think about our own lives and their edges. We cannot think about ourselves without thinking about Jay; and we cannot think about him without being intensely self-reflective.

What decisions will we, Jay's surrogates, make about Jay at the end of his life? What decisions did we make about our parents, who predeceased us? Did we have to agonize about whether to treat them or not, or how to treat them if indeed we decided to be aggressive in intervening to postpone their deaths? What were the principled grounds for our decisions? Were we more concerned with them (and their suffering) or with ourselves?

The decisions we made about others may well reveal what we want for ourselves. Have we executed advance directives, Last Wills and Testaments, health-care powers of attorney, living wills, and the like? What do we provide in them? What do they tell us about ourselves and thus about how we will decide, if we can, about Jay and about how others should decide about him? Has Jay executed similar instruments? Was he competent to do so? Was he fully informed about the consequences of his decisions? Did he act voluntarily? Or was he acting at our behest, relying on us, as he has always relied on us?

"Suffering" Disability. At the core of these self-reflective questions lies our sense of how we "suffer" from disability and how the person who "has" the disability "suffers" from it (Hauerwas, 1986). Do we "suffer" because we are uncomfortable in Jay's presence, in the presence of disability; is disability in Jay and others who have it so disquieting? Or do we "suffer" because Jay is suffering. If the latter, the question is: why is he suffering? Is it because of the disability? Because he is being treated and has always rejected the tubes, bandages, and re-

straints that accompany a treatment? It could well be: disability can bring real pain for which there is no palliation, just as wounds and their treatment are insufferable to him.

If we suffer because Jay disquiets us, then the cure lies within ourselves, within our ability to shape our own responses to him and his disability. The cure has to lie within our ability to shape our own responses to life and its inevitable disabling consequences on others and on ourselves.

Let us assume that we "suffer" because we have not come to grips with the existential meaning of disability, with the significance of Jay's life. In that case, it may also be that we have not reflected enough on our own lives, on how we would want to be treated or intervened with when we are at the edges of life. To ask ourselves to do so when we are considering Jay and our own children or other family members who have disabilities is to ask us to be existentially self-reflective. It is to ask us how we "suffer" our own lives, how we understand them.

Who we are, what we aspire to be, and how we want to be treated or intervened with, then, is a measure of how we think Jay and others who have disabilities want to be and how they want to be treated or intervened with, given that they cannot express those sentiments effectively.

If we want a dignified death, to be spared the consequences of being kept alive through all means, then that is probably how we want Jay and our children with disabilities to be dealt with. We impute to them the same values, the same choices, as we exercise for ourselves. We see Jay as ourselves; our empathetic imagination identifies him with us and us with him. We act accordingly, doing "unto" and for Jay what we would have done unto and for ourselves. That "golden rule" invokes ethical, if not theological, models; it may also be consistent with various cultural norms; and it trumps the other models.

RIGHT REASONS, WRONG RESULTS; RIGHT RESULTS, WRONG REASONS: THE PARADOX OF SURROGATE DECISION MAKING AND THE LESSONS OF HISTORY

Paradoxes. The word "paradox" means a tenet that is contrary to received opinion. It refers to an argument that apparently derives self-contradictory conclusions by valid deduction from acceptable premises. Thus, when making decisions about Jay at the edges of his life, we expect a particular result to flow from our decisions, yet we obtain a result we did not anticipate. For example, we have been taught to expect some "bad" consequences from disability ("institutionalize Jay" was the soon-after-birth advice), yet there is a powerful body of first-person and third-person narratives that teach us that Jay offers us inestimable, positive gifts (Turnbull & Turnbull, 1978). We have been taught to expect little from Jay and others with disabilities, yet we find that he and they exceed our great(est) expectations. What is the paradox at the edges of life? What do we expect but not receive?

To answer that question, let us remember the quandary that attends any decision about life at the edges. The quandary is that our choice for ourselves may be denied to our child with a disability. Our autonomy—our models for our own lives—may be denied to our "Jay" relatives.

We ourselves may seek and assert a right to manage our physical and emotional pain, to palliative care, and to receive hospice services. We have come to expect them. Yet those same palliatives and hospice may not be available (at appropriate levels) to people with disabilities. We may want to die with dignity, but the person with a disability may not be allowed to die with dignity.

How is this so? It is so because we or others may exercise all the right reasons for treating Jay and intervening against Jay's death, but still reach the wrong result, which is to deny him death with dignity. We may so surround his and others' lives with so many rights, protections, and advocacy against the "dying of the light" that we deny them the end that we ourselves want and want for them (even after we acknowledge and account for all conflicts of interest).

We may also reach the right result for the wrong reasons. Despite our instincts to let Jay stop "raging," we may keep him alive artificially, heroically and extra-ordinarily, and this may be the "right" result. Or we may not keep him alive as long as we can.

Whatever result we reach, we do so because the constitutional, ethical, or "model" approaches compel us to reach it. In short, we may have to use those approaches that "the collective we" have ordained even though we personally do not want to use them, and in using them we may reach the right result: a person lives or does not, and yet we are not intellectually and spiritually content with the result.

The paradox is that we get what we do not expect or necessarily want, either because we did or did not do the right decision-making, the right reasoning. How do we come to this result? Why does it obtain? Why the paradox?

History and Its Lessons; Models and Their Constraints. In our discourse about what we want for Jay and ourselves, we must reflect on the history of how the "collective we" have regarded and dealt with people with disabilities. Our history is a mixed one.

It begins with compassion (the original meaning of the asylum). It proceeds to exploitation. It teaches us the wisdom of Trilling's admonition about altruism: the objects of our pity soon become the objects of our study and then the objects of our coercion (Trilling, as cited in Rothman, 1980).

In response to our coercion, our history then proceeds to rights (both negative and positive, rights against being exploited and rights to the "good life" to a "quality of life"). We apply the public law model, indeed, the rights sub-model, in order to create a different life for Jay than he would have obtained had we not generated new rights and implemented old ones.

We also rely on the human capacity model. We face life at the edges with the presumption that we can enhance Jay's capacity to live (if not also to live well). We adhere to the rights model and do all we can to adhere to his rights, so we apply the technological model and its imperative in service to our rights and human development models. We say, Jay has a right to live; we have the means to prolong his life; we therefore have a duty to do so. Right reasons, wrong results? Do these models prevent us from doing what our instincts and hearts tell us are right actions? Are we constrained by the rights, human development, and technological models?

So we ask, What lies beyond rights? What is the post-rights paradigm? What role is there for a sense of "rightness?" Dare we return to "compassion?" On what other models may we rely? On what principles?

MODELS AND THEIR LIBERATING ELEMENTS; BEYOND RIGHTS AT JAY'S EDGE OF LIFE

Models for Living and Dying. We must dare to talk about a post-rights paradigm, to find a place for "rightness" and compassion. Indeed, we can do just that because we have established rights for those with disabilities (and corresponding duties for ourselves) and equal rights for ourselves. It is not that Jay has no rights and we have no duties. He has plenty of rights, and we have plenty of duties. Beyond rights and the public-law model, however, there are other models that have shaped our lives with Jay. We have acknowledged the cultural model, especially by asserting that disability is a social construct and by bringing to bear all sorts of rights and technology to improve the fit between Jay and his world. We also have lived consistently with the ethical-theological model, especially by claiming that public (legal) rights rest on moral (ethical) grounds and by helping Jay acquire a faith in our God.

When Jay Turnbull comes to the end of his life, I hope that we will not constrain ourselves by a rights model that denies him the very means for living well as he is dying, the very dignity of leaving this life, that I want for myself and that I am absolutely certain he wants for himself.

It is not just that Jay believes in Heaven and God and "Baby Jesus" and believes that those in his family who have died are in Heaven with God and Baby Jesus. It is not just that he applies a theological model to his life and the death of others.

Nor is it just that Jay has opted for a life that is rich in quality, that is surrounded and enriched by social connections, that is supported, protected, and advocated for by a large host of surrogate decision-makers, by his circle of friends, his community, and his amici.

Living as the Warrant for Dying. No, it is more that we know what Jay wants. His life gives us a warrant, a justification, for decisions that are existential in the gravest sense of that word, in the sense that there is the bed on which he lives and dies and the grave into which he will be laid and the question: what is the significance of Jay's life? Jay is a *Cruzan* and a *Saikewicz*; he is precisely the person around whom there is "trust," not just rights. In both cases, the courts trusted someone to make a decision for the person with a disability. Yes, the cases took the stage as a play about rights; but they concluded as lessons about trusting someone to act compassionately. That was their final curtain.

Trust, then, is an element of our decision-making, a necessary one that is hard to grapple with: whom do we trust, and how much trust do we place in that person? Whom does Jay trust? How implicitly, how thoroughly?

Jay is the person whom we his parents have entrusted to others during half of his life; we entrust him to others even as we contemplate our own pre-deceasing, our own departure before he comes to the edge of his life/dying.

More than that, and consistent with the autonomy principle, we have trusted Jay to make decisions about the essence of his life, about with whom, how and where he will live, work, and have social (and deeper) connections.

And, in terms of Jay's circle and community, Jay and we have trusted others to respond to him–to be his protectors and his advocates, his amici. And in trusting him and others, he and we have no choice but to continue to trust him and others, even after we die. That is the consequence of living in community with others, of acknowledging the "first-edness," the primacy, of family and of having a wide sense of family as encompassing people in Jay's community of living.

So we look to such principles as dignity, family as foundation, and community to guide us, and we rely on cultural and theological models more, at the edges of life, than on other models.

I am libertarian to the core on this matter. If I or Jay's family and circle/council/community are unable to make the decisions at the end of his life, then of what value has been the rights-creating life I have lived and from which Jay has benefited? I may have helped create rights but I may also have denied Jay the dignified death that my mother, father, and father-in-law had and that I want for myself and that other members of Jay's (and my) family want for themselves and for me and, most significantly, for Jay.

We must guard against our history, but knowing it allows us to do so. Jay and we together have developed a life for himself/him that is based on rights and also on trust and compassion. We trust ourselves not to exploit Jay in his life and we dare not exploit him in his dying.

Beyond Rights; Trust and Compassion. So, in the end, we can move beyond rights to what is right. We can move beyond the Jay's claims that he should not be discriminated against because of his disability (a negative-rights posture) and even beyond his claims to effective interventions (a positive-rights posture). We can move beyond those claims to a claim that Jay makes, which is that we rely on his trust in others and on their compassion-driven response. We can move to a model of cultural, ethical, and theological decision-making that trumps the models of human capacity and public (rights) decision-making.

The trajectory of Jay's life–his history as part of the disability community history–is now such that we are in and must be allowed to continue to live and die in the post-rights era. Rights, yes; trust and compassion, yes. They are not necessarily inconsistent and when the end comes for Jay we must look more to trust and compassion, to the culture Jay and we have created around him and to the ethics and theology that are so much part of his life, than to rights.

Leave us–his family, his circle, his community–alone to make our own decisions in our own ways, knowing how Jay has chosen to live and having made his choices a reality for himself and us.

Trust us with Jay, for Jay trusts us with himself. He always has and he always will, even unto the end.

REFERENCES

American Association on Mental Retardation. Policy Statement: Quality of Life. Washington, DC: American Association on Mental Retardation (position paper adopted by Board of Directors of American Association on Mental Retardation, May 28, 2002).

Child Abuse Prevention and Treatment and Adoption Act, 42 U.S.C. Sec. 5106a.

Cruzan v. Director, 497 U.S. 261 (1990).

DeShaney v. Winnebago County Department of Social Services, 489 U.S. 189 (1989).

Elk Grove Unified School District v. Newdow, 124 S. Ct. 2301 (2004).

Federal Register, Vol. 50, pp. 14878-14901, Apr. 15, 1985.

Hauerwas, S. (1986). Suffering the retarded: Should we prevent retardation? In Dokecki, P.R. and Zaner, R. M. (eds.). Ethics of dealing with persons with severe handicaps. Baltimore: Paul H. Brookes Publishing Co.

Principles of Treatment of Disabled Infants (1983). Statement signed by officers of American Association of University Affiliated Programs, American Association on Mental Deficiency (now, Retardation), National Down Syndrome Congress, National Association of Children's Hospitals and Rehabilitation Institutes, Spina Bifida Association of American, TASH: The Association for Persons with Severe Handicaps, ARC-US (Association for Retarded Citizens of the United States), American Academy of Pediatrics.

Superintendent v. Saikewicz, 373 Mass. 728 (1977).

Stowe, M.J., Umbarger, G.T., & Turnbull, H. R. (2004, but in press for 2005). Connections among the core concepts of health policy and the core concepts of disability policy. *Journal of Disability Policy Studies*.

The Arc (2002). Policy Statement: Quality of Life. Silver Spring, MD: The Arc (position statement adopted by Congress of Delegates, The Arc of the United States, November 9, 2002).

Thomas, D. (1957). *Do not go gentle into that good night*. Collected Poems. New York. New Directions.

Trilling, L., quoted in Rothman, D. (1980). Conscience and convenience: The asylum and its alternatives in progressive America. Boston: Little Brown.

Troxel v. Granville, 530 U.S. 57 (2000).

Turnbull, H.R. (ed.) (1978). Consent Handbook. Washington, DC: American Association on Mental Deficiency.

Turnbull, H.R., & Turnbull, A.P. (eds.) (1978). Parents speak out: Views from the other side of the two-way mirror. Columbus, OH: Charles E. Merrill Publishing Co.

Turnbull, H.R., Beegle, G., & Stowe, M. J. (2001). Core concepts of disability policy affecting families who have children with disabilities. *Journal of Disability Policy Studies*, *12(3)*, 133-143.

Turnbull, H.R., & Stowe, M. (2001). Five models for thinking about disability: Implications for policy. *Journal of Disability Policy Studies, 12(3),* 198-205.

Umbarger, G. T., Stowe, M.J., & Turnbull, H.R. (2004, but in press for 2005). The core concepts of health care policy affecting families who have children with disabilities. *Journal of Disability Policy Studies.*

Vacco v. Quill, 521 U.S. 793 (1997).

Washington v. Glucksberg, 521 U.S. 702 (1997).

RESPONSES
TO "WHAT SHOULD WE DO FOR JAY?"

What Should We Do for Everyone?
Response to "What Should We Do for Jay?"

Angela King, MSSW

SUMMARY. The *Last Passages* project has been discussing end-of-life care for people with developmental disabilities for the past three years. The project has gathered best practices information and disseminated it through training, publications and websites. This response reflects many of the discussions, policy recommendations and philosophy of care developed by the *Last Passages* project. We believe we must insure that each person, regardless of their disability, has the opportunity to make end-of-life care choices, or have them made by family members and/or friends whom they trust, and that those choices be respected and supported by health care providers and the legal system. *[Article copies available for a fee from The Haworth Document Delivery Service: 1-800-HAWORTH. E-mail address: <docdelivery@haworthpress.com> Website: <http://www.HaworthPress.com> © 2005 by The Haworth Press, Inc. All rights reserved.]*

Angela King is Program Director, Volunteers of America, 2002 Deer Path, Arlington, TX 76012.

[Haworth co-indexing entry note]: "What Should We Do for Everyone? Response to 'What Should We Do for Jay?'." King, Angela. Co-published simultaneously in Journal of Religion, Disability & Health (The Haworth Pastoral Press, an imprint of The Haworth Press, Inc.) Vol. 9, No. 2, 2005, pp. 27-31; and: *End-of-Life Care: Bridging Disability and Aging with Person-Centered Care* (ed: Rev. William C. Gaventa, and David L. Coulter) The Haworth Pastoral Press, an imprint of The Haworth Press, Inc., 2005, pp. 27-31. Single or multiple copies of this article are available for a fee from The Haworth Document Delivery Service [1-800-HAWORTH, 9:00 a.m. - 5:00 p.m. (EST). E-mail address: docdelivery@haworthpress.com].

Available online at http://www.haworthpress.com/web/JRDH
© 2005 by The Haworth Press, Inc. All rights reserved.
doi:10.1300/J095v9n02_02

KEYWORDS. End-of-life care, *Last Passages*, aging and disability, developmental disabilities, hospice and palliative care

In reviewing the article, "Edges of Life and Cognitive Disability," I was impressed by the philosophical and ethical principles that are reviewed and discussed. The article offers a very complete discussion of the principles and legal definitions that guide decision making in end of life care. However, in the midst of all these noble ideas, Mr. Turnbull comes back to rely on the values of family, compassion and trust in making end-of-life care decisions for his son. Surely, this reliance is reflective of our internal moral compass and our human desire for love and community. I agree that the values of family, compassion and trust are the ultimate considerations in end-of-life care decisions, regardless of an individual's disability.

During the past three years, Volunteers of America has conducted a project called *Last Passages*, disseminating information regarding the best practices in end-of-life care for people with developmental disabilities. One of the outcomes of this project was identifying and convening a national advisory board, made up of parents/family members, disability advocates, medical professionals, ethicists, and others who have a passion for insuring that people with developmental disabilities have access to end-of-life care planning and choices. Many of the principles identified in Mr. Turnbull's article were discussed at length at advisory meetings and included in written materials that were developed for training purposes. Certainly, the individuals who participated in the *Last Passages* project would, wholeheartedly, support the principles identified in this article and would agree that end-of-life care decisions are best made by family members and friends who have known the individual throughout his/her lifetime and who can relay the wishes and desires of the individual based on their years of knowing and supporting.

Mr. Turnbull's article begins with an explanation of medical principles that are used to guide end-of-life care choices; the choice of appropriate health care, defensible medical judgment and the right and duty of health care treatment. In the context of the article, Mr. Turnbull refers to physicians who have known his son Jay throughout his life. These physicians have treated Jay for many years; they respect him and recognize his family members and their right to assist in making decisions for their son. However, while Mr. Turnbull's article makes an excellent presentation for the end-of-life care decisions his son may need, it does not recognize the issues we confront when an individual's life has been unstable, when their health care providers have changed numerous times, when there are not family members and/or friends to assist with decision-making and when the person's access to community has been limited by circumstance and discrimination. End-of-life decision-making is not a single event that occurs when faced with a critical illness, but, rather, an on-going series of choices, based on life experiences, family and friends' support systems, as well as health issues. Our philosophy is that individuals with developmental disabilities should be allowed and encouraged to articulate these choices, throughout the course of their lives, so that their wishes can be respected.

Safeguards have been developed that include ethic committees, public guardians, case law and regulatory procedures, all intended to protect the rights of an individual with a disability, an individual who may have been unable to express their choices for end-of-life care. Often we find, that individuals with developmental disabilities have been left out of the ebb and flow of life, shielded from the death of parents or other family members, excluded from funerals and memorials and not allowed to develop ways of coping with grief. No one has ever asked the person with disabilities, or given them an opportunity to express their choices regarding their own burial, funeral or end-of-life care. The first step in providing quality end-of-life care is involving the person, over the course of time, in discussions regarding death; what they believe about the end-of-life and supporting choices that reflect those beliefs. Discussions regarding end-of-life care should not be a formalized one-time event, but rather part of a natural discussion that takes place over time. Opportunities for learning should be maximized and individuals with developmental disabilities should be allowed to participate in their culture's rituals around death, including funerals, remembrances and other activities that occur during the natural course of one's lifetime. In the article, Mr. Turnbull refers to Jay's pastor, which is a testimony to Jay's involvement with a faith community. Too often, individuals with developmental disabilities have no faith community and have not been allowed to develop or express their beliefs regarding what happens after death. At the end of life, faith is often a great comfort, a source of hope and a foundation for the belief that our "soul" transitions to eternity. Without this connection we are left with the sterile application of ethics and regulations denying the recognition of the individuality of the person with a disability, their belief system and their choices.

While we all recognize the rights of individuals with developmental disabilities to exercise choice regarding end-of-life care, we have often failed to provide individuals and their families with the training and support they need to make these choices. Additionally, we have failed to educate the health care community, and at times the general public, regarding the differences in facing a terminal illness and living with a chronic disability. Several advocacy groups are, with good reason, expressing a growing concern with discussions of end-of-life care that preclude the use of life sustaining technology that many individuals with severe disabilities use every day. Decisions must be made with a pro-disability attitude. We must be clear in our advocacy for individuals with developmental disabilities that each person has the right to life, despite the level of their disability. Every person has the right to choose curative care, even in the face of a dismal prognosis. The right to high-quality palliative care should also be fully extended to individuals with developmental disabilities who choose this end-of-life treatment option. Healthcare providers must recognize and value the difference between disability management and prolonging the end-of-life. We believe that people with developmental disabilities must have access to the full range of end-of-life care options that we want for all our citizens. Working together, in a pro-disability movement, we can insure that our system of care, including long term and acute care options, fully support an individual's choice.

Certainly family and/or friends are the foundation of the choices in end-of-life care decision-making. Each of us must consider who will make choices for us when we are not able to speak for ourselves, due to declining health, injury or illness. We must trust that our family and/or friends will speak for us protect us, and insure that our life ends in a manner that reflects how we have lived, what we value and the choices we have expressed. The sad fact is that many individuals in our society reach the end of their life without family or friends to express these choices. It is these individuals we must also be concerned about when developing the parameters of end-of-life care choices. Throughout the country, there are many individuals with disabilities who have grown up in circumstances where family members have abandoned them or perhaps, preceded them in death, leaving no close relative to provide a historical perspective of their life. We still have numerous people in our service "system" who have moved from place to place, institution to community, service provider to service provider as we have struggled to improve the lives of people with disabilities. We believe that the full range of choices available in a community should also be available for people with developmental disabilities. Services such as hospice, home health, family support, health care and spiritual comfort should be available to individuals with developmental disabilities, regardless of where they live. The right to die at home should include supportive living residences and group homes that often provide services to people with developmental disabilities.

Faced with a lack of family and/or friends, people with disabilities are often in the position of having decisions made for them by public guardians or services providers. While well-meaning and often long term supporters of the person, guardians and service providers have been reluctant to make decisions regarding end-of-life care for people with disabilities. Reasons for this reluctance have included legal barriers, conflicting medical opinions and perceived ethical conflicts. However, I would offer the opinion that an unspoken barrier to assisting with end of life care choices for people with disabilities relates to the issues that Mr. Turnbull raises, the foundation of family and the intimacy of end-of-life care decisions. It is an emotional connection that often determines choices made in end-of-life care. It is a human connection, based on respect for the individual who is dying, for their life and their choices and an emotional bond of love and compassion.

I agree, as Mr. Turnbull indicates, that end-of-life care decisions should be left to family and friends and that these decisions should be made on the basis of compassion and trust. Given this belief we must act to insure that all people with disabilities have people in their lives who can be trusted to care for them, not just within a legal framework, but with an emotional connection. For those individuals who lack that connection, we must continue the safeguards based on ethical principles as stated in the article. There may always be a need for ethics committees and I am certain there will continue to be legal battles regarding end-of-life care choices. However, I am hopeful that by involving individuals with disabilities in community, by supporting family connections, and by encouraging the development of long-term friendships, we will come to rely more on family and friends and less on courts and committees to determine end-of-life care choices for people with disabilities. To have the ability over the course of our lives to communicate our choices and to have those choices honored by people who love us, by people we trust, by people who understand our faith beliefs and value the life we have lived, that is what we all hope for when facing death. A person with disabilities should expect nothing less.

The Challenges of Living and Dying Well: Response to "What Should We Do for Jay?"

Genevieve Pugh, MA, NHA

SUMMARY. This response reviews the universal goal for a good end of life and explores the unique challenges faced by individuals with disabilities and their families and friends when confronting issues of death and dying. The foundations necessary for the unfolding of good end-of-life planning and the roles played by individuals and their advocates are critical elements of this review. *[Article copies available for a fee from The Haworth Document Delivery Service: 1-800-HAWORTH. E-mail address: <docdelivery@haworthpress.com> Website: <http://www.HaworthPress. com> © 2005 by The Haworth Press, Inc. All rights reserved.]*

KEYWORDS. End of life, developmental and intellectual disabilities, advance directives, quality of life

Rud Turnbull provides us with a clear and comprehensive exploration of the legal, moral, ethical and social issues surrounding end-of-life planning for a person with intellectual disabilities. Once again, Rud, Jay, and their family have been generous in sharing their lives and in do-

Genevieve Pugh is Director, Black Mountain Center, 932 Old US 70 Highway, Black Mountain, NC 28711.

[Haworth co-indexing entry note]: "The Challenges of Living and Dying Well: Response to 'What Should We Do for Jay?'." Pugh, Genevieve. Co-published simultaneously in Journal of Religion, Disability & Health (The Haworth Pastoral Press, an imprint of The Haworth Press, Inc.) Vol. 9, No. 2, 2005, pp. 33-35; and: *End-of-Life Care: Bridging Disability and Aging with Person-Centered Care* (ed: Rev. William C. Gaventa, and David L. Coulter) The Haworth Pastoral Press, an imprint of The Haworth Press, Inc., 2005, pp. 33-35. Single or multiple copies of this article are available for a fee from The Haworth Document Delivery Service [1-800-HAWORTH, 9:00 a.m. - 5:00 p.m. (EST). E-mail address: docdelivery@haworthpress.com].

33

ing so, have made the important issues of end of life real and approachable.

For all of us, the core issues can be defined as what we want at the end of our lives and who can and should be empowered to make the decisions that will affect how closely our experience matches those wishes and desires. Most people, when asked, say that they would like to die at home, as comfortably as possible, with friends and family around them. In fact, that happens for a relatively small number of people. Nor do most people die traumatically. Many people experience the end of life in hospitals and with interventions and treatments that may prolong life but do not change the ultimate outcome. We are a culture that has difficulty letting go. We are blessed with health care providers whose training has focused on healing and saving lives. It is in this context that much work has been done to educate Americans about their options for advance directives and to encourage conversations with doctors and family members to insure that written plans and knowledge of individual wishes will ultimately drive the care decisions made at the end of life. In spite of the efforts to educate, many people have not had these conversations, made these choices and communicated them clearly.

Unfortunately, it is distressing to see how often this reluctance to let go is not extended to people with disabilities.

In reading "What Should We Do for Jay?" and in considering the emphasis in our culture on having a good death, it is possible to forget that for many people, especially those with disabilities, the foundations are simply not in place for the unfolding of good end-of-life planning. Many people with disabilities more likely do not have a primary health care provider who knows their history or has a relationship that allows an appreciation of the meaning of their lives. Unfortunately, they have little or no routine medical care and the local emergency room provides their care when they are ill. The people who know them best and love them most may not be empowered legally or otherwise to speak on their behalf. Rather, the decision makers may be involved more by biology, agency responsibility, or by virtue of being on call in the emergency room on the particular night that a need for decision making becomes most critical. Under these circumstances, the factors to consider in decision making take on an increased sense of urgency. Rather than planning based upon a lifetime of knowing a person well, beneficence may be more a function of a health care provider or well meaning guardian's personal beliefs and values. Often, the phrase "quality of life" becomes a prominent feature in this process and the risk exists that the distinction between a living a life with a disability and having a terminal condition becomes blurred. One person's life of suffering is another person's good life. This slippery slope becomes even more precarious when it is forgotten that the individual is the determinant of his or her perception of quality of life, not those who are seeing the situation through their own values and circumstances.

The ultimate goal for a good end to life is universal and the ability to realize this goal should not be compromised by disability or economic status. All people should have the opportunity throughout their lives to communicate their wishes and desires about how life will end and to expect those expressions of intent to be honored. People with disabilities should have full access to a complete array of aggressive medical treatments and should have options for palliative care and supports at the point in life that they choose those services. When individuals do not have capacity to give consent directly, the laws that protect them should not deny those who know them best the legal right to speak on their behalf.

How do we move forward so that all people have something closer to the experiences of Jay and his family? We do that by working to insure equal access to health care. We do that by continuing to affect legal process and public policy so that a balance is achieved between protection and access to a full range of options. We do that by educating individuals with disabilities and their families, friends, guardians, and health care providers. We ensure that education and communication occurs before we are faced with imminent decision making about end-of-life care. Much work is necessary to insure that all health care is provided in concert with the wishes of each individual and in ways that insure that people with disabilities experience the same potential for responsive care as others in our culture. In the end, prepared and empowered individuals will have the greatest control over end-of-life care.

Euthanasia and Disability: Comments on "What Should We Do for Jay?"

Hans S. Reinders, PhD

SUMMARY. In his paper, Turnbull raises an important but often unrecognized point, which is that there are certain limitations to what rights can do for us. He introduces the notions of "trust" and "compassion" in order to indicate the kind of limitation he has in mind. While I am sympathetic to his general position at this point–there are certain concerns in the ethical domain that cannot be properly addressed by the notion of rights–I think the author owes his readers a more explicit explanantion about what it is that rights cannot do in the particular case he presents us with. Thinking about this case, Turnbull finds himself trapped in a paradox, which leads him to believe he must move beyond rights claims. The paraadox, as he describes it, is that if we stick to rights claims in order to protect people with disabilities against various kinds of discrimination in the context of health care, they might end up in a situation where neither they nor we want them to be. *[Article copies available for a fee from The Haworth Document Delivery Service: 1-800-HAWORTH. E-mail address: <docdelivery@haworthpress.com> Website: <http://www.HaworthPress.com> © 2005 by The Haworth Press, Inc. All rights reserved.]*

Hans S. Reinders is Willem van den Bergh Professor of Ethics and Disability, Vrije Universiteit, Amsterdam, The Netherlands.

[Haworth co-indexing entry note]: "Euthanasia and Disability: Comments on 'What Should We Do for Jay?'." Reinders, Hans S. Co-published simultaneously in Journal of Religion, Disability & Health (The Haworth Pastoral Press, an imprint of The Haworth Press, Inc.) Vol. 9, No. 2, 2005, pp. 37-48; and: *End-of-Life Care: Bridging Disability and Aging with Person-Centered Care* (ed: Rev. William C. Gaventa, and David L. Coulter) The Haworth Pastoral Press, an imprint of The Haworth Press, Inc., 2005, pp. 37-48. Single or multiple copies of this article are available for a fee from The Haworth Document Delivery Service [1-800-HAWORTH, 9:00 a.m. - 5:00 p.m. (EST). E-mail address: docdelivery@haworthpress.com].

Available online at http://www.haworthpress.com/web/JRDH
doi:10.1300/J095v9n02_04

KEYWORDS. Ethics, end of life, intellectual disability, euthanasia, rights, family, physician assisted suicide, death with dignity

THE CASE

So what is the case the author is reflecting upon? The case is about his son Jay, a grown-up man of 37 with an intellectual disability and a chronic heart condition. It is the combination of these two facts about Jay, presumably, that induces his father to think about what will happen when Jay is at the end of his life, and his parents are no longer there. The question Turnbull thus arrives at is: Who will decide what to do, by what standards will they decide, and under what procedures?

This is a real question because, as the author informs us, Jay has no legal guardian. His parents have always supported him as his natural guardians, acting as his surrogates, seeking what is best for Jay, with his assent. Furthermore, Jay's health care is assured by a number of private contracts between his parents and their health care providers to which Jay is "the third-party beneficiary of a contract" while he is "the direct beneficiary of the services." This state of affairs indicates that when his parents are no longer there to occupy this role, there is indeed an open question as to who will replace them, and what the terms of Jay's health care provisions will be.

Facing his family's future, the author takes it to be certain that Jay will outlive his parents and, on that assumption, projects the following scenario. At a given point in time, Jay's medical specialist certifies that he is within six months of his death, while there is no reason to dispute his judgment. Jay has not been declared "brain dead" or "organ dead." Furthermore, Jay is not in state custody. Assuming that his son is in a state of unconsciousness, there is no way of asking Jay what he wants, in that situation.

The last assumption in this scenario is crucial, of course. Up to now, Turnbull tells us, Jay has been consulting with his physicians, but it is questionable, his father asserts, "that he fully understands the nature of their treatment," including the effects of certain medications. But at the same time we are told, although much later in the discussion of the case, that Jay has even executed several "advanced directives." Turnbull also asserts more than once that he is sure Jay knows what he wants, and that his family knows it too. There are apparently different sides to the matter of Jay's competency when it comes to his ability to make up his own mind on what should happen in the last stage of his life.

Hence the author's question: What will those who replace Jay's parents decide, and, on what grounds will they decide?

THE ARGUMENT

The author proceeds to answer his question in a quite laborious manner by listing a wealth of material that somehow has a bearing on the case: sixteen principles of various kinds, followed by an equally impressive number of procedural rules and models. One striking aspect of Turnbull's presentation of this mixed bag of legal, ethical, and professional principles is that he is not very elaborate in explaining the normative order between them. We need to know how the various principles should be prioritized in case they come into conflict with one another. No justification of a particular course of action–legal, ethical, or otherwise–upon which conflicting principles have a bearing, will ever succeed, logically speaking, when there is no normative order of their priority. That such is the case in the situation at hand is evident in my view.

Turnbull develops a convoluted argument with quite a few loose ends and unresolved tensions. But apart from this, what he wants to say is in the end quite clear, and, I should add, important. As Jay's father, he has been a disability rights advocate most of his life, but now that he faces the final stage of his own life he worries about what will happen to his son, particularly when his chronic cardiac condition will make him fatally ill. In his reflections on this projected situation, he anticipates that the success of the advocacy movement may obstruct the possibility of dying well for his son. The unexpected outcome may well be that in the end Jay will not be permitted to die in a dignified way.

> *How is this so? It is so because we or others may exercise all the right reasons for treating Jay and intervening against Jay's death, but still with the wrong result, which is to deny him death with dignity. We may surround his and others' lives with so many rights, protections, and advocacy against "the dying of the light" that we deny them the end that we ourselves want and want for them.*

The possibility of dying with dignity for his son is the author's main concern. Now, the question is what it would mean for Jay to die with dignity. Unfortunately, Turnbull never addresses this question explicitly, either conceptually or normatively. However, there are a number of signs in his text that indicate what he may have in mind; for example, when he expresses his fear that at the end of Jay's life his physicians may take it to be their duty to use "any technology that has proven to be effective," or when he suggests that the quality of Jay's life may eventually be "enhanced by its termination," or that "physicians may fear that their decision will be challenged in the courts as inconsistent with professional practice." Each of these remarks seems to indicate that what he has in mind is a decision that Jay's life is not prolonged at all costs. Accordingly he asserts that the courts as well as The Arc and AAMR have accepted the legitimacy of "quality of life judgments when life is inevitably ending." I take such statements to suggest that what Turnbull has in mind in speaking of dying with dignity is, conceptually, the option of terminating life-sustaining treatment for Jay for reasons of quality of life, and normatively, that Jay's family ought to be permitted to decide when the moment to stop such treatment has arrived in case he is no longer conscious (irreversibly comatose).

It is with this understanding of what dying with dignity means in this case, presumably, that the author comes to express his concerns regarding the mechanisms of rights and protections for people with disabilities enshrined in the law: "We say, Jay has a right to live; we have means to prolong his life; we therefore have a duty to do so. Right reasons, wrong results?" The answer to this rhetorical question is clear, at least for Turnbull. We must move beyond rights to allow proper decisions in this case, for which he appeals to trust and compassion as the key notions for an alternative approach. "Trust" in this connection implies that Jay's family (i.e., his sisters and friends) ought to be entrusted with making decisions about Jay's death. "Compassion" implies that we should not let Jay become a victim of his own rights. But again, this interpretation is conjecture on my part because the author does not make explicit what he means when he speaks of dying with dignity. Nor does he make explicit what he has in mind in talking about "trust" and "compassion."

QUESTIONS

Before addressing the general point Turnbull makes, I will raise a few questions about specific details of the case that I think are puzzling. As was indicated already, there is some ambivalence in the author's account of Jay's competency. Turnbull claims that the principles of "liberty and privacy" include, among other things, "to have Jay's judgment be exercised by us for him." If this does not mean that Jay has expressed an opinion on the matter, what does it mean? Considering the legal validity of statements by the person whose death is under consideration, Turnbull says that even when Jay was not able to make those kinds of statements, there still would be the evidence from his behavior: "his behavior is communication; both oral and written communication." What oral and written communication? Furthermore, his parents "have trusted Jay to make decisions about the essence of his life, about with whom, how and where he will live, work, and have social (and deeper) connections." Since I would not know what higher level of competency one could possible have, one cannot help wondering what is wrong with Jay's competency. Anyway, the question remains where is Jay in all this? If Jay has been competent to create advanced directives, why is he incompetent to be involved in talking about the case his father ponders? Why not have an advanced directive on the foreseen scenario?

But maybe I have misinterpreted the claims about Jay's competency because they were not literally meant to say that Jay is capable of making judgments. Maybe the author only wants to claim that he knows what Jay wants because Jay has "almost always" assented to the decisions his parents made for him. Maybe Turnbull's main point in this regard is to say that it would be very hard for others to understand what Jay wants, but that this is different for his family. They know what Jay wants because they know Jay. This much weaker interpretation of Jay's competency would explain why his father states:

> *If we want a dignified death, to be spared the ignobling consequences of being kept alive through all means, then that is probably how we want Jay and our children with disabilities to be dealt with. We impute to them the same values, the same choices, as we exercise for ourselves. We see Jay as ourselves; our empathetic imagination identifies him with us and us with him. We act accordingly, doing "unto" and for Jay what we would have done unto and for ourselves.*

When I read him correctly, this is the heart of the matter when it comes to Turnbull's moral reasoning. He thinks that Jay's family should be permitted to make decisions with regard to Jay's death on the basis of the Golden Rule. That is to say, having shared their lives with Jay's according to their own values, they want to be entrusted with decisions about Jay's death on the basis of these same values. Even though Turnbull is aware of the fact of cultural variety–implying that occasionally we may be worried about other people's values–he nonetheless believes that the Golden Rules "trumps" other models of decision-making. This explains what he means when he confesses to be "a libertarian to the core on this matter." People ought to have a right to make decisions in the case at hand on the basis of their own values.

With regard to this claim, however, much more needs to be said to make it morally convincing. Turnbull argues that the Golden Rule suggests "ethical, if not theological models" of decision-making. Well, it certainly does.[2] But as the literature on the Golden Rule makes abundantly clear, the mere fact that I want a given action done to myself is hardly a sufficient *moral* reason to say that I should do the same action to someone else. It is arguably not even a sufficient reason to do so when the other person agrees. Both the other person and myself may have been socialized with a morally despicable set of values.

THE LAW

Apart from the moral reasoning in Turnbull's argument, there is in this connection also a question about its legal aspects. Before raising it I should say that it does not stem from extensive knowledge on my part of the "law of the land" (i.e., the American constitution and case law); instead they stem from how Turnbull presents what he takes to law to be.

As indicated, he claims that family decision-making is acceptable in the case at hand, for which he appeals to the principle "family as foundation," which the author lists as an ethical principle. It is stated it as follows:

> *Family as foundation acknowledges that for Jay, as for minors and many adults who have cognitive disabilities, his family is the core social unit in his life and the ultimate decision-maker because it has transmitted values that Jay is presumed to adopt; there is no evidence that he has lived a life that is counter to those values and that therefore his family's values should not be imputed to him.*

Where does this principle leave the author when it comes to the legal aspects of the case? Consider the ruling of the US Supreme Court as Turnbull presents it: decisions regarding the continuation of life-sustaining treatment in cases of terminal illness cannot be left to the discretion of individual citizens and their families because these matters, though in the realm of their private lives, "are issues that state legislatures must determine." With this ruling the Supreme Court apparently denies the family the role of the "ultimate decision-maker" in cases such as Jay's in the sense that it cannot be left to their discretion on what values they want to make the decision in question.

To sustain his position, Turnbull appeals to two famous court cases, known as *Cruzan* and *Saikewicz,* in which the legitimacy of decisions on continuing life-sustaining treatment was at stake. The author suggests "in both cases, the courts *trusted someone* to make a decision for the person with a disability." But as he has demonstrated already, the courts laid down explicit rules for proper legal decision-making, including rules with regard to what kind of evidence is and is not acceptable. Decision-makers are not trusted in the sense that the decision is left to their discretion. On the contrary, they are bound by strict rules of evidence so that if their decision violates these rules, the courts will overturn it. The ultimate decision-maker is the law, this is to say, at least from a legal point of view

Furthermore, even if it were true that in *Cruzan* and *Saikewicz* the courts permitted quality of life judgments, as Turnbull claims, that still does not justify the family as ultimate decision-maker. As Turnbull presents these cases, the courts only permitted legal *representation of the person's views* by a surrogate. That is to say, surrogate decision-makers have to produce strong evidence to prove that they know the decision that the terminally ill person would have made had he or she been competent. The courts did not allow the judgment on the matter to be grounded in his or her family's values.

Whatever these legal considerations amount to, Turnbull's account of the law indicates that he thinks he can make the legal case. "Jay is a *Cruzan* and *Saikewicz,*" he claims, which presumably means that what is ruled in their cases should also hold for Jay. If the courts permitted life-sustaining treatments to be terminated because the views held by these persons themselves were convincingly represented, they should eventually permit the same in Jay's case. But now another puzzling question arises. If the author is right in claiming that Jay's projected case is similar, then it is unclear why legal rights to equal protection of persons with disabilities should be counter-productive at the end of Jay's life. Under the required circumstances the law would allow the option of eventually discontinuing life-sustaining treatment if sufficient evidence of Jay's own judgment on the matter can be produced. Since the author claims to know what Jay wants, which he infers from the fact that Jay's "behavior is communication; both oral and written communication," it does not seem impossible to produce the kind of evidence the courts require. Furthermore, since there are no legal obstructions to getting Jay into palliative care or hospice care, it is unclear which course of action that the author or his family may eventually prefer is legally blocked. The law *as Turnbull reads it* does apparently not condemn what he wants for his son.

If so, the question is how we are to read the author's claim that we have to move "beyond rights." If the rights of people with disabilities enshrined in the law do not prevent Jay's family to make decisions regarding his death–as his father claims–it seems that the argument that we need to think "beyond rights" must have a different aim. It cannot be that the law gets in the way of dying with dignity in Jay's case because the father claims that Jay's case is similar to cases where the courts have decided in favor of terminating life-sustaining treatment. Instead, I read Turnbull as intending to open up the discussion on a highly sensitive issue in the community of disability rights advocates, of which the author has been an active member of this community for most of life. The issue is euthanasia for persons with an intellectual disability.

EUTHANASIA AND DISABILITY

I take it, then, that Turnbull's main objective is to open up a discussion about euthanasia in the field of intellectual disability. Coming from a country in which euthanasia is accepted by the courts under certain conditions, it may be helpful to make a few observations on its development.

One observation is that the history of euthanasia in The Netherlands clearly shows the reality of a "slippery slope" in how people think about it. Philosophers often have criticized "slippery slope" arguments as invalid, because it is not necessarily true that in legalizing voluntary euthanasia we will end in a situation where people are killed against their will for presumably benign reasons. But this criticism is valid in only a very limited sense, because it only reads "slippery slope" arguments as prospective. I read them differently, namely in retrospect. What I then see in my own country is that until the mid 1990s the discussion was restricted to what Americans call physician-assisted suicide. The Dutch even invented a definition of euthanasia for themselves, which was "ending a patient's life upon his or her explicit and repeated request." This indicates that the debate at that time was about whether the principle of autonomy should include autonomous decisions regarding one's own death. Most people in The Netherlands felt that it should but only under strict conditions. What has been legalized is ending a patient's life only upon that patient's explicit and repeated request. This was the most important restriction.[3] As the Dutch insisted again and again, there could be no question of killing vulnerable people such as the severely disabled without their consent.

However, since 1994–when the political compromise for this limited permissibility was forged–the debate has shifted. Now the issue became what to do with human beings who face a horrible death, which question was–and still is–particularly raised with regard to severely disabled newborn infants. The restricted definition of euthanasia was not formally abandoned, of course, but now the question of "dying well" was again on the table. In retrospect, the Dutch are discussing cases that they proclaimed ten years earlier were not part of the debate.

A further observation is that in recent years the euthanasia debate has gradually entered the field of intellectual disabilities. That does not mean that there is an increase in the actual practice of euthanasia in this field.[4] However, if not the practice, the debate is clearly growing. Given my work in ethics and disability, I am regularly requested by service providers to address the issue of "what to do at the end of life" because "our staff is asking for guidelines." Many service providers offering residential services are busy drawing up protocols and procedures to that end. The ones I have seen make explicit that actively ending a person's life is not permitted. The motive may be ethical ("we think it is wrong"), or legal because, as it stands, euthanasia is still on the penal code so that professionals and their organizations that take responsibility for an act of euthanasia still face the possibility of a trial.

But also here things are changing, particular in the area of neonatology. The courts seem to be moving in a direction where the condition of terminal illness replaces the patient's request as a necessary condition. The interesting thing is that this appears to be similar to what Turnbull seems to be promoting. Doctors consult with families in case death is unavoidable and the patient is seriously suffering. In cases where there is an agreement that it is in the child's best interest to die, life-sustaining treatment may be discontinued.[5] The case has to be fully documented and must be reported to the district attorney. In cases where the guidelines have been properly followed, the doctor may be acquitted.

Given these observations, rather than joining the debate on where to go from here, I would rather make the admittedly odd suggestion to reconsider the merits of the notion of a "taboo" on this subject. If there is anything in the Dutch discussion on euthanasia that appalls me, it is the complacent self-confidence that misleads my fellow countrymen in thinking that our deaths can be the proper subjects of public regulation. The problem of euthanasia in the case of children with severe disabilities is not new. What is new is the idea that we need a law to regulate it.

People in the past have frequently faced the same question of what to do with severely suffering infants and they have found their way with it, while keeping the doubts and agony among themselves. Was that necessarily worse than what we now have?

The obvious rejoinder from the disability rights movement will be to remind me of the fact that keeping it silent is exactly what happened with, for example, involuntary sterilization. Rightly so, but my point is not that passed practices were preferable. It is rather that I do not believe that public regulation will allow us to fare much better. I do not believe, that is to say, in controlling the practice of euthanasia by means of the law. Particularly not when we take Turnbull's libertarian position. On that position, any regulation that limits our freedom to make decisions for ourselves must appear as arbitrary: "your ethics against mine." Once they are seen in that perspective, legal limits to individual freedom do not last long in liberal democracy.

BEYOND RIGHTS

But of course, nobody will let me get away with the suggestion to reconsider the merits of taboos in this connection. The point of bringing it up is not to make a practically feasible suggestion, however. For a long time I have believed that whatever else one may think about it, the Dutch development had at least this advantage–that the issue of euthanasia is openly discussed. I am no longer convinced that this is an advantage. At any rate, many people in The Netherlands involved in decisions about ending a patient's life–doctors, families, and patients– think the process of dying and helping people to die is not an area for the law to interfere with. Until the present day there is continuing worry by legal authorities that cases of euthanasia are underreported, this in spite of its clearly regulated legitimacy.[6]

In the end I believe, therefore, that what one thinks of these matters depends indeed on trust. How much do we trust other people in making decisions and acting in accordance with their own values, and with regard to which decisions, and with regard to whom? In cases like the one Turnbull puts before us, any argument based on the principle of "family as foundation" must depend on the tacit assumption that the values of one's family are all right. Only on that assumption is it true that the values Jay's family lives by may be imputed on Jay, and that they are a justifiable basis for moral decision-making. But taken in a general sense, the assumption as such is questionable, as Turnbull probably would accept. There have been appalling cases of abuse of people with disabilities, even within their own families, to mention only one thing.

Can people be entrusted to proceed in a morally justifiable way when making decisions about how their loved ones die? Sometimes I am sure they can. Sometimes I am equally sure they cannot. This is probably why most of us think there needs to be a law in order to uphold the distinction between the two, since we do not necessarily trust other people's ethics, that is to say, we think there needs to be a law that stops them from doing what we think is wrong, even when they think it right. However, while we have our doubts about other people in this respect, at the same time most of us tend to think that we can be trusted in the discretion of our own judgment.

Curiously enough, Turnbull finds himself in a similar position. He wants Jay's family (Jay's sisters and friends) to be trusted with the decision-making, but at the same time he wants them to be guided by the decision-making framework that he himself has developed. Trust is apparently an ambivalent matter when the edges of life are at stake.

In one thing Turnbull is very right, in my view, and that is his claim that in the end how we think about the death of a loved one is primarily dependent on what we think about our own death. Put generally, how we think about the lives of persons with intellectual disabilities is primarily a reflection of how think about ourselves, more than it is anything else.[7] In this connection, Turnbull indicates that he knows how he wants to die. I am not so sure that I do. I may have some idea of what I want now for then, but I have no idea of what I then want when the time is there. I have been at the bedside of a few loved ones who were dying. From that experience I have learned that whatever redeeming aspects there were in how they died, they were entirely dependent on our openness to be receptive to them. That is, in the end, my worry about Turnbull's argument. I don't think death is a matter of our own control. Rather than knowing *what to do* in the kind of situation he reflects upon, I would rather reflect upon *how to be* in that situation.

Must we go beyond rights in thinking about how we perceive dying well, either for ourselves or our loved ones? No doubt we must, but not in order to enlarge the moral space for people to make decisions of their own, particularly not in view of the conflicting norms and values in our society with regard to disabled lives. In this respect I am much more reluctant than Turnbull seems to be. In thinking about disabled lives we must go beyond rights for a very different reason. True insight into what my life is ultimately about will help me see what someone else's life is ultimately about, disabled or not. The more we understand our own limitations, and see through the illusions of "controlling our lives," the more we will see how much our lives are like theirs, notwithstanding the many differences. Who of us, after all, really believes themselves to be competent with regard to their own deaths?

NOTES

1. For an extensive argument in support of this claim, see Hans S. Reinders, "The Good Life for Disabled Citizens," *Journal of Intellectual Disability Research*, Vol. 46, part one, January 2002, 1-5.

2. See Hans S. Reinders, "The Golden Rule between Philosophy and Theology," in Alberto Bondolfi, Stefan Grotefeld, Rudi Neuberth (eds.) *Ethics, Reason, and Rationality* (Münster: LIT Verlag, 1997), 145-168.

3. Apart from the explicit and repeated request, the guidelines required the condition of "unendurable suffering," a second opinion from another doctor, and a well-documented decision. Importantly, the condition of terminal illness was not included, mainly because the Dutch Medical Association rejected it for its impracticability. Legally, "terminal" would require a time limit (3 days, 1 week, 2 months?). Doctors, it was said, have no way of predicting the moment of death with reliable certainty.

4. As the last social scientific survey showed in 1998, ending the lives of people with intellectual disabilities with terminal illness was hardly ever practiced (only one case had been found). At any rate the incidence was significantly lower than in other areas of health care.

5. The so-called "Groningen-protocol" that was in the media recently, reporting 22 killings of terminally ill babies since 1997 in The Netherlands, apparently goes a crucial step further, which is to end the patient's life with a lethal injection. The cases involved "extreme *spina bifida*." The legal prosecution did not result in charges in cases where four "unofficial rules" were met. The child's medical team and independent doctors must agree. There is no prospect of improvement and the pain cannot be eased. Parents give their consent. The life of the child must be ended in the correct medical way.

6. The doctors involved in the "Groningen Protocol" have stated that the problem of underreporting was the main reason for bringing their knowledge of the facts out in the open. "The babies are there but we were never allowed to talk about them," said doctor Verhagen of Groningen University Medical Centre.

7. See on this point Hans S. Reinders, *The Future of the Disabled in Liberal Society: An Ethical Analysis* (Notre Dame IN.: The University of Notre Dame Press, 2000), 159-209.

The Writing on the Wall . . . Alzheimer's Disease: A Daughter's Look at Mom's Faithful Care of Dad

M. J. Iozzio, PhD

SUMMARY. From a reflection on the challenges of providing care for a person with Alzheimer's (AD) disease, a daughter's look at mom's faithful care asks questions of AD disabilities, of virtues, and of the necessary and uniquely human prospects of interdependent/Trinitarian modeling existence. The first question considers the pathology of AD and other complicating health conditions. The second question explores the development of virtues, such as flexibility, stamina, humor, fidelity, and self-care that may enrich care-giving. The third question suggests that the current model of US healthcare inadequately finds justice for persons marginalized either by their unwelcome dementia or isolating care-giving. *[Article copies available for a fee from The Haworth Document Delivery Service: 1-800-HAWORTH. E-mail address: <docdelivery@haworthpress.com> Website: <http://www.HaworthPress. com> © 2005 by The Haworth Press, Inc. All rights reserved.]*

KEYWORDS. Alzheimer's disease, virtue, theological anthropology, interdependence, healthcare, justice

M. J. Iozzio is Associate Professor of Theology, Barry University, Miami Shores, FL 33161.

[Haworth co-indexing entry note]: "The Writing on the Wall . . . Alzheimer's Disease: A Daughter's Look at Mom's Faithful Care of Dad." Iozzio, M. J. Co-published simultaneously in Journal of Religion, Disability & Health (The Haworth Pastoral Press, an imprint of The Haworth Press, Inc.) Vol. 9, No. 2, 2005, pp. 49-74; and: *End-of-Life Care: Bridging Disability and Aging with Person-Centered Care* (ed: Rev. William C. Gaventa, and David L. Coulter) The Haworth Pastoral Press, an imprint of The Haworth Press, Inc., 2005, pp. 49-74. Single or multiple copies of this article are available for a fee from The Haworth Document Delivery Service [1-800-HAWORTH, 9:00 a.m. - 5:00 p.m. (EST). E-mail address: docdelivery@haworth press.com].

49

Every now and again I hear my mother say "poor guy" in reference to my father who has Alzheimer's disease. The saying disturbs me because it suggests that the experience of Alzheimer's disease impoverishes him. I do not think of either of my parents as being impoverished and not simply because they do not want for essential needs. Rather, my parents are comfortable, and my father doubly blessed, with faithful care. Mom's remark points, however, to a kind of poverty that betrays a philosophical and theological commitment to autonomy and independence, which has been unambiguously ingrained in the ethos of the western psyche since the Enlightenment. As I watch and help my mother with my father's personal and hygienic care as well as the care that is her attentive presence to him, I find myself mindful of one thing: my father's dignity. Surely, Mom's remark addresses this same concern. And I want to reframe her thinking from sympathy over an inability to wash, dress, feed, toilet, and entertain himself to an appreciation of a new way to be with him and he with us. Fortunately, every now and again I also hear my mother say "marvelous, thank you for letting me help you" and "what a good guy" in reference to his cooperation and his own "thank you" to her for this or that kindness.

Nevertheless, I am troubled by the assignment of indignity that seems to follow so closely upon the experience of a loss of control over one or another bodily and/or mental functions. If dignity is a quality or state of being worthy of esteem or respect,[1] the assignment of indignity begs the question of the criteria that redress to autonomy alone cannot satisfy. Infants and children are very often 'out of control' and yet few among us would deny them the dignity that belongs properly to them as members of the human family. Some people with disabilities also lack control of their speech, of their limbs, and/or of their bladder and bowel,[2] yet few among us today would dare deny any rights accruing to persons with disabilities as distinguished and dignified members of the human community. Rather, occasions of a loss of control and the likely accompanying need of help from others provide criteria worthy of human flourishing: when we tend in particular to the bodily needs of another we demonstrate a very deep respect for the person and a faithful care for the material in which the person lives, and moves, and has being. Thus, despite the historical associations of the care of bodies to women's work and the accidental experience of my mother's care for my father in this way,[3] care of another's body challenges the intellectualizing tendency of dualism and the elevation of things spirit over matter. Any loss of bodily or mental control does not, by itself, remove or reduce the intrinsic dignity abiding in my father or everyone else.

My father's condition invites both critical reflection and reappraisal of the ways in which my mother and our extended family interact and relate with him and with one another. The relation with my mother and the family of parental and patriarchal authority that my father held has changed. That change has occasioned my thinking about being together over and against my thinking about separate, even disparate and unrelated, lives–interdependence over autonomy. Relations, I have come to believe, characterize the ground of human flourishing far better than autonomy, the hallmark principle of western notions of liberty and of bioethics discourse. Relations, I have come to understand, both distinguish and unite us in ways that demand a commitment to change and grow ever more perfectly into the image and likeness of God who is revealed in the relations of the Trinity.

Lovers, once intimately attuned to each other's rhythms, find themselves negotiating life's blessings and curses with a stranger. Children, having managed adult relationships with their parents, find themselves in reversed roles mothering or fathering them. Sisters and brothers, after fiercely asserting their uniqueness, find themselves holding desperately to the old familiar. Not suspecting the moment when I am no longer recognizable to my lover, parent, brother, friend, I am caught off guard by their unknowing. How do I remain faithful to them when they question, because of Alzheimer's dementia, who I am?

Alzheimer's disease (AD) arrived in our family unwelcomed, and lingers. The disease exacts an unrelenting toll on patients and caregivers, challenging accommodations and acceptance, patience and presence, health and well-being, which toll ends only with death and a modicum of relief. AD destroys those parts of the brain that control memory, leading to impaired motor, language, and reasoning skills, contributing to the impaired function of all organ systems. AD engages caregiving in formal and informal settings, leading to qualitatively important interactions between patient and the caregiver as moral agent. This article examines the unknowing dementias that AD exhibits in the patient and the child-like dependency to which Alzheimer's patients degenerate, and the co-extensive response of caregivers. AD may be unwelcome but its presence in our families requires sustained attention. Without this sustained attention we may succumb to the feminist and liberation theologies' recognition of harms from the counter-intuitive disposal of the easily oppressed and marginalized–the socially unproductive demented elderly and their seemingly equally unproductive caregivers.

In this article I will consider the experience of my family–especially those of my mother as primary caregiver and father as afflicted–as we manage the daily work of Alzheimer's patient care. Besides the pathological progress of the disease, I will explore some of the key virtues that care for the Alzheimer's patient requires: flexibility, stamina, humor, and, above all, fidelity and self-care. The present literature in bioethics on AD focuses on autonomy and beneficence. However, in this article I shift the focus away from the critical setting and abstract ethics committee meetings, where the hallmark bioethics' principles garner participants' attention and practitioners target problem solving. I am convinced that the focus of discussions on AD belong in the home care setting, where the problems are multitudinous and persistent and where caregivers are sometimes only just getting by. Critical ethical reflections on AD are more properly directed to the relationships between intimates that are now compromised by dementia.[4] The daily work of AD patient care locates our ethics in being with and doing for the other in need–those qualitatively important interactions between persons.

The reasoning used in this article follows a casuistry dependent on an Aristotelian-Thomistic virtue rather than a deontological principlist ethics. This casuistry requires a careful analysis of the contextual features that define experiences and set them apart from others. Like a feminist ethics that attends to the defining circumstances of the particular here and now, the classical yet neglected casuistry of the late medieval period[5] attends in sometimes disarming detail to those same circumstances. Although traditionally used to settle cases of conscience or doubt where a projected course of action conflicts with standard procedures, I use casuistry here for its method of analysis and not for its expected resolution of a dilemma. AD is not a dilemma; it is a condition that inflicts its debilitating effects on human beings–mothers, fathers, sisters, brothers, lovers and friends–and demands an appropriately human response to their needs to live and die well.

First, I will consider the dependency of human relationships and of the uniquely compromising relationships of informal caregivers to their loved ones, who are now patients. This consideration includes the diagnosis and prognosis of AD as well as the nature of the relationships between patient and caregivers and between primary and other supporting caregivers. Second, I will order those relationships and focus on the relationship between the primary caregiver, the patient, and the primary supporting relationships of care (my mother, father, her sisters and brothers, my brothers and sisters and their children, my cousins, and me and my husband). This ordering will clarify the needs of the caregiver as a moral agent as well as those of the patient without sacrificing the integrity of either by maintaining the concentric spheres of concern and support of related others. Third, I will examine the experiences of caring for an intimate other who no longer recognizes the relation, who no longer knows the stories, and who is a different self still in need of intimacy. This examination will explore the ethical responsibilities that distinguish enduring relationships. This distinction returns to the Alzheimer pathology and to the anthropological nature of interdependent existence as generically compromised and yet uniquely designed for human flourishing.

These three considerations are hinged to certain theological insights that will distinguish the three parts of the article: human beings are created in the image and likeness of a triune God, we are all fundamentally free (however compromised our intentions and choices may be), and the poor and marginalized deserve an abundance of the world's resources and grace.

Key conclusions will turn on faithfulness and the virtue of fidelity. While a corrupted version of this virtue may isolate the primary caregiver from social outings given the persistent needs of the Alzheimer patient, fidelity becomes a virtue when it is mediated by prudence and balanced with justice and self-care.[6] The virtue of justice, giving to others their due qua human, calls us to attend to those who are marginalized because of their isolation. That call to justice points to the anthropological basis of these reflections, which is itself rooted in a teleological vision of the good life as radically dependent on both intimate and communal relations and love. Further, with deliberate attention to the unpredictable course of relations with a person who has AD, I suggest that the current system of healthcare in the United States offers little support for the care of the chronic infirmed. For too long this system has relegated domestic care to the socially disadvantaged. Fidelity to them directs this redress.

A THEOLOGICAL ANTHROPOLOGY OF RELATIONALITY

My thoughts on relationality and dependence arise from recent experiences my husband and I have had with my immediate family, each of which concern the daily work of care for an elderly parent whose health is already compromised by diabetic neuropathy, kidney failure and confirming symptoms of AD. I was struck by the radical dependence for so many routine activities of my once commanding father upon my mother during our visits to one another's home. From personal hygiene and choice of clothes to reading books and entertaining, he requires vigilant help, which she obliges patiently. As a daughter I am challenged to reflect upon the reality that is the newly unpredictable life of my mother as primary caregiver and father in desperate need of care as well as of my brothers and sisters, my aunts and uncles, my cousins, me and my husband, and our children. And as a theologian I am challenged to see how this reality can be reconciled with the revelation of God in the Christian understanding of creation, the Incarnation and the Trinity.[7]

The Christian revelation and doctrinal truths of creation, Incarnation, and Trinity provide the foundation for my theological reflections on dependence by challenging a presumably normative Western liberalist and absolutized autonomy.[8] Instead of a pseudo collection of autonomous selves that arise from the theorizing of philosophical liberalisms, I am suggesting that the radical dependence that is found in these Christian truths belongs to the very meaning and end of human life and that, in the end, autonomy betrays human flourishing. We are radically dependent upon our parents, families, and friends (or some other responsible persons) from the moment of our first breath and all through our formative years (we remain dependent on a host of others for all manner of life-critical needs: the farmer, transporter, and grocer reveal only one very small set). And we are radically dependent upon God for, among manifold graces and love, the blessedness of everlasting life. Radical dependence challenges the ultimately isolating ends of the de rigueur absolutized autonomy of our post-modern times.

Consider these doctrinal truths. By creation humankind is born into mortal life for a return to eternal life; in the person of Jesus of Nazareth humankind incarnates God where God is one with us as one of us; and with the Trinity humankind realizes unity in diversity, the necessary preconditions of relationships and love. These doctrinal realities—of creation, Incarnation, and Trinity—reveal an unabashed dependence required of (even seemingly autonomous) individual as well as communal existence. The creation of the world needed, i.e., depended upon the Creator; and, as God created this world, God became dependent upon the manifestation of this creation in order to reveal Godself to us.[9] The Incarnation needed, i.e., depended upon, by God's own will and choice, human flesh; God became dependent on Holy Mary and all her ancestors for the material of the Son. The Trinity needed, i.e., depended upon relationality if God is to be revealed in physical time and space in the Creator, in Jesus, and in the Holy Spirit; God becomes dependent on the Divine Persons for God's very work of revelation. Dependence is neither a bad word nor a bad idea when viewed from the perspective of the interdependent union and communion of the Divine Persons revealing our God.[10] And, based on these doctrinally-confirming realities of dependence, I propose that dependence is neither a bad word nor a bad idea when viewed from the perspective of the interdependent nature of human existence.

I have surprised myself in moving from a christological toward a trinitarian model for understanding the nature of human existence.[11] Yet this move strikes me now as obvious. In Christology thinking about human beings turns on the birth, death, and resurrection of Jesus–the gospel good news and God's revelation in flesh to the world. In trinitarian theology thinking turns on the relationship between, of, and from God the Creator, God the Word, and God the Spirit. The Trinity and the Christ of the Trinity are of necessity, by the terms of the revelation to humankind, a reality that exposes relationships. Of course all discussions of Christology must at some point address the revelation of Jesus the Christ as the Second Person of the Trinity. Likewise, all discussions of the Trinity must at some point address the revelation of the triune God in the Person of the Incarnate Word. I am arguing that the theologically explicit relationship model of the Trinity presents a paradigm for the interdependent nature of human existence, with its distinct and ever-increasing number of individual human beings, all of whom are created in the image and likeness of this triune God.

The theological grounds for this anthropological relationality are rooted in the interdependent nature of human existence imaging the triune God and demonstrate the morally important features of this kind of interdependence for human flourishing. Thomas Aquinas, and following his thought the *Catechism of the Catholic Church*,[12] offers a discussion of the Trinity that builds on this philosophical category of relations and dependence within relations. Once the philosophical foundations are set for relationality within the Trinity, the paradigm for human relationality arises logically. As one of the defining characteristics of humankind, relationality presents a key to the means of happiness that, like the radical dependence revealed to us within the Trinity, defies liberalized autonomy. This happiness is characterized especially by human flourishing, both in this life and in the life to come. And flourishing can only happen concomitantly and as a result of real dependency on others. The moral imperatives of interdependence return us to the concerns of care for persons whose health is compromised by dementing illness.

Relationship in the Trinity

The divine persons are distinguished from each other only by the relations that exist in the order of the divine essence.[13] Aquinas' deliberate use of the qualified 'only' suggests to me an opening for my inquiry into the interdependent nature of divine and human existence. As with any scholastic theologian, Aquinas chooses his words carefully and purposively. After discussing the procession of the divine persons, from the Father in the Word and in Love, he takes up the philosophical category of relations in respect of God. These relations are one of a series of categories following the metaphysics of Aristotle, which Aquinas attributes to God so that he may distinguish within the Trinity the distinct persons Father, Son, and Spirit.

The particular kind of relation that exists in God is a real relation vs. a logical or comparative relation, which is a relative opposition that includes (shall I venture to say depends upon) distinction.[14] 'Only' real relations are determinable in regard to internal processions in God: those relations derived from the action of the intellect, i.e., the procession of the Word, and those relations derived from the action of the will, i.e., the procession of Love. Hence, in God the real relations are generation, filiation, and spiration.[15] These relations direct Aquinas' thought toward the subsequently necessary examination of the Divine Persons in common and singly. In this examination he finds that as real relations exist in God, as well as between God and creatures, these relations must of necessity belong to Persons, who signify what is distinct in a particular rational nature. For example, I am one person distinct from all other persons, who are all nevertheless human beings sharing the essence of human beings, and it is only by distinction that I can be related to other persons. In God, since distinction is derived likewise by relations, those relations signify the substantial essence of God.[16] "In God the hypostasis is expressed as distinct by the relation."[17] Thus, for Christians, God is one nature in three distinct persons by way of relation. The dependence of the Father to the Son and to the Spirit is of necessity the manifest revelation of the real relations between the distinct persons of the Trinity;[18] we do not know the Trinity in any other way.[19]

From a trinitarian perspective then relations and relationality ground the interdependence of real being. God is three persons in an intimate and perpetual relation that is characterized by and realized only through interdependence. When considered from the perspective of the Trinity, interdependence and dependence then ought to appear more attractive to liberal strongholders of absolute autonomy and extreme independence.[20] If God wills to be dependent, as the Trinitarian distinction of persons requires for the purposes of revelation to humankind, then how can independence be a hallmark achievement for human individuals and why is dependence cast in so bad a light? God's achievement through the dependent relations of interdependent relationality is creation, Incarnation, Love. Human achievement through independence, on the other hand, is non-existent.[21] If God willed independence for Godself, revelation would not be necessary; subsistent nature requires nothing and is therefore dependent upon nothing, not even itself.[22] However, once God acted it was then that generation, filiation and spiration proceeded and was brought forth; interdependence reveals God essentially and in the manifest world of which we are a part. Further, God's interdependence causes the creation, the Incarnation, and Love to flourish. Revelation thus indicates God's flourishing as unity in diversity. From a trinitarian perspective then the interdependent relationality of the real being of God creates humankind in God's own relationally interdependent image.

Human Relational Interdependence

Human beings are rational bodies, composed of multiple and multiply dependent faculties (the will, reason, and sensory perceptions, to name a few) that are indispensable to the individuality–to the distinction–of the persons they reveal. This distinction is the beginning of the fullness of the revelation that human beings are created in the image and likeness of the triune God; this distinction is the beginning, too, of the fullness of the revelation, the summum bonum of human flourishing, toward which human beings are called: to be related intimately with the triune God.[23] Only by being a distinct person can any human being enter into a relation with another and only by being related to another can any human being become a distinct person. Further, only by being in relation can these persons flourish individually and together. Thus, just as the Trinity reveals relational interdependence, human beings, as distinct persons sharing a common nature, reveal the relational interdependence required of personal identity and solidarity in the human community.[24] Rational embodiedness distinguishes each person from all other persons and from the other creatures in the kingdom; and interdependent relationality unites, both because and in spite of distinctions, all those sharing the form and purposes of the one human nature.[25] Interdependent relationality, like Trinitarian relationality, becomes a key for the anthropological presuppositions of human flourishing.

This key to the anthropological presuppositions of human flourishing provides concrete evidence of the proper ends and ways to be human. If the telos of human life is at all discernable, then the rational embodied nature of human existence has its purposes, by the force of interdependence, in the happiness that is characterized by the flourish of relationality that results in union with others and with God. The popular absolutized notions of independence and autonomy, on the other hand, subvert this telos of human flourishing by idealizing superhuman individualism. But the laws of nature and grace, which identify the purposes of human life as communion-love, support the proposition that neither woman nor man can live independently or alone . . . for long. The laws of nature and grace recall not only the inclinations to preserve and perpetuate life but these laws recall also the inclinations to have companions and search for truth together.[26] Interdependence and relationality become the necessary preconditions of human flourishing by attention to the needs of the basic physical, intellectual, emotional, social, and spiritual growth and development of every distinct person. Further, without relations human beings would not know the love–the fundamental exchange of "me" for "us"–that becomes the foundation for the flourish of the relationality that yields to the happiness of union with others and with God.[27] This love returns to the ultimately defining relational character of the human image of the triune God. Interdependent relationality thus defines the ways that human beings are in the world.

Further, the love that characterizes the happiness of union–the flourish of relationality–may be understood in respect of both a natural and a supernatural end, both of which ends, moreover, depend for their realization upon the being and the help of others. Like the triune God, whose very being is unity in diversity, human beings attain the end that is the happiness of union only through being in the relationality of diversity. In addition to the happiness of being in relation, the happiness that results with the help of others may take the form of the physical, intellectual, emotional, social and spiritual support of family, friends, teachers, and social organizations in conjunction with the form of the superabundant grace freely offered to us by God. I could not know of what the happiness of this life consists without the interdependent relationships that characterize my particular life nor could I merit the supernatural happiness of everlasting life or even know of its existence without the grace of God.[28] Both of these realities (natural and supernatural happiness) reflect the interdependent and relational nature of human existence that is characterized by the help that comes from others and from God. Further, the natural and the supernatural are interdependent, interrelated, and fully integrated;[29] free will and grace together lead human existence into purposive life. Thus, the achievement of an ever greater freedom of distinct persons united with others and with the triune God who shares the divine life with us becomes the happy purposive end of the human flourish of relationality, the summum bonum, the natural and supernatural happiness that is proper to humankind.

MORAL CONSIDERATIONS OF INTERDEPENDENCE AND THE COMPROMISES OF AD

Contrary to the choice-critical issues that formal bioethics engage, interdependent relationality points to the ordinary day-to-day care of a person with a debilitating dementing illness. This change of direction in the discussions over appropriate care for and decision making with the person who has AD challenges the preconditioned responses to what we might do given the principles of autonomy, beneficence, non-maleficence and justice. Instead of a more clinically-centered model of casuistry that decides competency for the purposes of critical decision making capability, for example, AD raises an other-centered model of casuistry. Responses from this critique engage ambiguity, intersubjectivity, and the varied contexts of the lives of real people and their families.[30] Responses to discussions over appropriate care for an AD patient demand attention to the patient and the caregiver as well as the relations that support this dependent reality.

The diagnosis and prognosis of AD are arrived at only hesitantly by most medical practitioners. This hesitancy stems from the lack of diagnostic tests to confirm the presence in the brain of the tangles and plaques around the nerve cells, finally indicative of AD, that retard communication from one neuron to another. Confirmation of AD is difficult to ascertain; previously, only post-mortem brain autopsy provided definitive diagnosis. Today, when dementia is suspected, a series of evaluations and laboratory tests may be conducted.[31] Starting with a conversation to detail a person's history, thorough physical and neurological exams reveal both the current state of health and differential data on nervous system functioning. From these initial exams other possible causes of a person's dementia may be discounted. A series of blood chemistry, thyroid functioning, lumbar puncture, and activities of daily living batteries can confirm an irreversible dementia. CT scans or MRI may reveal structural anomalies and changes in the brain associated with the neuron tangles and plaques of AD. Finally, recent studies suggest that mutations in certain genes, which may be identified through genetic testing, may mark a predisposition to or the presence of AD (65% late onset AD patients have APOE4, amyloid plaque molecule, at chromosome 19).

Like millions of other persons with dementia,[32] no absolutely definitive diagnosis of AD has been made of my father. Nevertheless, he is being treated for AD with a number of the drugs recently available to thwart the debilitating progress of the disease. Diabetes and the recent determination of significant loss of kidney functioning further compromise my father's condition.[33]

AD has compromised not only my father's ability to care for himself and for the relationships that he has nurtured through his lifetime, AD has also compromised my mother's ability to care for herself and for the relationships that she has nurtured through her lifetime. These compromises provide the context for the moral challenges of interdependent relationality. The content of those challenges involve not only the 'principle' issues of autonomy, beneficence, non-maleficence and justice, but these challenges involve also—and more difficultly and poignantly—the virtues of self-care, fidelity and humor, the expressions of ambiguous intersubjectivity.

Self-Determination, the Moral Key to Human Interaction

Let's return to Aquinas, for whom the beginning of the moral life arises in the exercise of the free will. Whether addressing the subject of the acquired virtues, grace, or charity, Aquinas recognizes the necessity of the freely willed intention and execution of the agent's choice. While on the surface this address appears to reinforce liberal notions of autonomy and independence, this intention and choice arise within persons who have been already shaped by the relationships that have thus far supported them, those relationships with family, friends, teachers, social organizations and God. Further, no one person arrives at a free decision without having first been provided with an object to be willed *and* an apprehension of the object *as a good*.[34] The exercise of free will then demonstrates the agent's understanding of the good as well as the community's degree of participation in helping to identify and define goods in the agent's moral life. Thus, to the extent that an agent succeeds or fails in correctly apprehending the good, so too has her community succeeded or failed in providing for her as an agent the skills necessary to apprehend and to will correctly. The interdependent nature of human existence is thereby characterized by the success or failure of this correct apprehension and willing of the good; the interdependent nature of human existence is thereby characterized by right orderedness in the individual exercises of free will in the rightly ordered lives of those in rightly ordered interdependent relations.

The self-determination that reveals this right orderedness requires a certain ability that, from the discussions preeminently entertained in the bioethics literature, is lacking in persons with dementia regardless of when it is confirmed.[35] However, compromised decisional capacity does not warrant exclusion of these persons on the part of paternalistic caregivers from the decision making concerns of the right and the good. Persons with compromising dementia demonstrate, through often non-verbal means of communication, an appreciation of the complexities that dementia brings to a relationship.[36] Rightly ordered interdependent relations engage the remaining physical, intellectual, emotional, social and spiritual capacities that empower those who are compromised.[37] The challenge for caregivers is to decipher the choices of persons with dementia in ways that honor their implicit determination as well as their natural rights to retain a place in the relationships that define them.

Rightly ordered interdependent relations return to the introductory reflections regarding my father and our family. The radical dependence that my father exhibits betrays a mortality as well as a disability over which he, like us all, has no control.[38] The response of my mother especially, and other members of the family as well, imparts an embrace of the interdependent nature of human existence that accepts this time of radical dependence. The challenge of this time for my mother, father, and family is to recognize the distinctly different degrees of dependence at both predictable and unpredictable times within the extended life of interdependent relations: as infants and young children, when illness or disease present, if pregnant, when disabled, and in advanced age. Nevertheless, if rightly ordered interdependent relations are to image authentically the interdependent relations of the triune God, they must accept the unity and distinction of persons that is constitutive of human flourishing. Even when the diversity of interdependence is compromised, as in the case of a person with dementia–or with childhood, with some other compromising illness or disease, or with some other disabling condition–the ongoing and deliberately uniting work of others with persons so compromised makes the relationality between them real relation. Rightly ordered interdependent relations strive to relieve the compromises of AD or ambiguous intersubjectivity through, among others, the virtues of self-care, fidelity, and humor.[39]

The Content of Faithful Care

The return to virtue, both in and out of the academy, continues apace.[40] This sustained interest suggests a discomfort with abstract conceptions of a-historical or a-contextual principles, which fail to attend satisfactorily to the challenges of caring for someone with debilitating dementia. Principlist ethics often lack the means to uncover the ambiguous contexts encountered in the day to day living with and caring for a person who has AD. With its emphasis on autonomy especially, principlist ethics would deem a patient with advanced AD or other forms of dementia incompetent. This determination, however, can devolve all too easily into a dismissal of the alternate patterns of communication that defy critical incompetence and that maintain the relationality between persons with dementia and those who care for and about them.[41] By contrast, virtue ethics can more adequately uncover some of these contexts and provide the subject matter for the content of that care; the virtues measure ways to be as well as what to do here and now that refreshes and supports relationality for myself and for the person who is in my care. Further, the virtues belong to the category of actions known as immanent operations; as such, they affect both the doing of a particular act and the agent's formation in the moral life. Virtues become the language of the content of moral discourse when that discourse engages moral agents and their growth in freedom as they journey from first breath to last. Many virtues come to mind as necessary for the quotidian care of a compromised other, but self-care, fidelity and humor figure prominently as key to successfully managing this particular interdependent relationality.

First, self-care is, by definition, self-regarding care of personal bodily and spiritual integrity. Among the traditional list of moral virtues, self-care would be associated either with or may reveal a more contemporary home for the virtues of temperance and fortitude.[42] Temperance is that virtue concerned with moderation in matters of physical health and well being, while fortitude is concerned with managing the routines as well as the unexpected and distracting hiccup in those routines of daily life. Self-care belongs to interdependent relations insofar as, from the discussion above on the Trinity and on human existence as well as from contemporary psychological studies, no one can be in union with another without a distinct sense of self.[43] My mother, above all others because of both the immediacy of and her proximity to the needs of my father, must be diligent in her exercise of self-care. She must attend to her own physical, intellectual, emotional, social and spiritual needs as a distinct person called to happiness and to be in union with her family, friends, social groups, and God. The insights from feminist ethics, AA/Al Anon and other Twelve-Step programs, and virtue ethics recognize the needs and necessary—but not narcissistic or self-deprecating—demands of self-care for growth in the moral life as a woman of virtue and as a human being reflecting the image of the relations between the distinct persons of the triune God.

My mother and I speak frequently and I am all too aware of her need for respite care that would provide re-grouping; respite easily squares with self-care time. In the mid-season of the progress of my father's AD she did not seriously engage the prospect of regular professional intervention but she made arrangements for Dad to go to a daycare center two days a week, with hopes that other days would soon be available. She didn't necessarily "do" much on those days, a fact that bears little affect on the effect of respite. Now that the AD and concomitant health demise have been determined, respite comes in the form of home health aides from hospice, the Veterans' Administration, the County Office on Aging, and a private duty contract. Hospice offers additional respite programs that include a 5-day maximum stay in a skilled nursing facility. Other ways in which she attends to her own needs include daily Mass, laundry and ironing (activities that employ her efficiency with satisfying pride), visits with her sisters, and communion visits to parishioners unable to attend weekly services, among others. In spite of these times away from the immediacy of caregiving, without her utilization of the benefits of professional intervention she would be unable to care appropriately for her own needs and to attend to my father's need of affection and physical care.

Second, fidelity provides content to the nature of intimate relations and is thereby self- and other-regarding. Among the traditional list of moral virtues, fidelity would be associated with justice but its arena of activity, because intimate, requires more circumscribed attention than justice provides. Fidelity reveals the uniquely intimate relationships of distinct persons in marriage, families, and friendships and is characterized by trust, honesty, concern, presence, and constancy to name a few. Fidelity belongs to interdependent relations as the appropriate realization of the procession—divine and human—of words and love. My mother and father have been faithful for 55 years,[44] a short time in comparison to the fidelity between the Divine Persons, but which time defines them in important ways as wife, husband, and parents. To not abandon their faithful relationality they must continue to love, honor, and respect one another in this sickness as they have done so previously through other trying times as well as in health and times less complicated. The demands of fidelity for this intimacy free the distinct persons of the relation for consummate union, imaging the union toward which human persons are uniquely invited to join–charity-love and lasting friendship with God. To disregard this intimacy because it is now compromised by dementia or by any other disability forgets, ignores, and/or disdains the 'compromise' that is radical interdependency. Recall, dependency is neither a bad word nor a bad idea and, when framed in the context of real relations, dependency constitutes human and divine existence. This kind of intimate interdependent union, whether with lovers or with God, requires the steadfast trust and security of fidelity. Further, this union foretastes the supernatural happiness of heaven while sustaining the happiness in regard to flourishing with the intimate other in our midst.

My mother and father have been living together more than twice as long as either of them lived in their natal homes. This life in common has distinguished them individually and as a couple by the nature of the influences of intimacy upon intimates. Intimates speak to each other in a language devised for the confidences of personal revelation, they touch each other gently and reassuringly, they play with a view to each other's pleasure. My mother and father speak the language of friends, lovers, and parents; they hold hands and hug; they laugh at the same jokes; they worry for their children's safety and happiness. But when AD compromises intimacy, fidelity demands remembering.[45] As long as my father lives, the work of my mother, brothers and sisters, niece and nephews, her sisters and brothers/my aunts and uncles, my cousins, my husband and me is to remember for him. We work to put him back together, to re-place him in our relationships, to remember his sense of self. Even as he continues to lose his sense of self, which has been bound by relationality to my mother and our family these many years, we are to remind him of his place among and with us. Even as the dementia of AD causes him to not know us we are to know him. And even as he barely resembles the man he used to be–commanding, decisive, large–he is still husband, father, brother-in-law, and uncle to us. Fidelity asks this much of us, that we remain with him even as he fails to remember us, abandonment is not an option.[46] The fidelity we image for him even now imparts an embrace of the radical dependence of interdependent relations that continues to search for human flourishing.

Third, humor mediates the gravity of the complex circumstances of human life with a view toward the hope that comes to us in the wake of time and infinity. While not numbered among either Aristotle's or Aquinas' virtues, humor seems a ready candidate as one of those qualities of the mind whereby we would live rightly and (although many have made bad use of humor at the expense of another's integrity) which would be used to relieve, by putting into relief, taking life (too) seriously.[47] Both Aristotle and Aquinas recognize that amusement fills a natural place in intimate and social relations. Aquinas, commenting on Aristotle, writes that "as [we] sometime need to give [our] bodies rest from labors, so also [we] need to rest [our] soul from mental strain that ensues from [an] application to serious affairs. This is done by amusement."[48] Humor makes it easy to caricaturize (and then reconcile and appreciate) the incongruities of our life-plans with the many unpredictable events, happy or tragic, of our lives.[49] Humor belongs to interdependent relations as the vehicle and the measure of acceptance of the vulnerability and the vicissitudes of life.[50] My mother has, for as long as I can remember, been surprised and delighted by the story telling of my uncle. Most of his best stories have to do with things that happened to them while they were younger and which offer a glimpse into their lives and their all-too-human foibles that breaks the seriousness and the tension of awkward moments and brightens the celebrations of family gatherings.[51] That any of us would lose the facility to tell and appreciate the stories would constitute a failure not only of a sense of humor but a failure too of an appropriate sense of humanity/humility and the grace by which we continue to live.[52]

Some people like my uncle are very good at telling stories and the rest of us just get by. When my mother tells a story she forgets many of the key details but the telling divulges her ability to find humor in herself and to laugh with others about herself. My mother's not taking herself too seriously stems from her comfort with her family and friends, faith in God's providence in these as other times, and trust that whatever comes her security is assured. To dwell for any length of time on the deteriorating conditions of my father's health, failing memory or mental acuity would serve neither positive growth in her moral development nor any positive contribution toward Dad's well-being. At face value few see the humor latent in human frailty in its most extreme with aging or disabling compromises; many see instead a life lost and no longer worthy of the affections or conversations or caresses indicative of qualitatively important interactions between persons in real relation.[53] But humor helps Mom and the rest of the family to cope with the frustrations of Dad's unknowing and moves him, because it is contagious, to join in the laughter about ourselves and reconciles him to us again. Humor reminds us that in spite of our sincerest efforts we all fail at perfection and we sin, and in appreciation of these truths and of forgiveness, we smile.

JUSTICE FOR CAREGIVERS

Once the caregiver of an intimate with AD is safely nestled "in place" social systems that would have previously provided opportunities for shared activities, meaningful interaction, and stimulation decrease. That much of the caring for persons with dementia is provided by their families, i.e., people with whom the patient has been intimate either by virtue of marriage, parenthood, as sibling or significant other, leads all too easily to an unintentional sequestering within the confines of the patient's home. This sequestering effectively isolates the caregiver(s) and patients from much needed support and social interaction. Further, inasmuch as these caregivers are more often than not women, a two-fold critique of this pattern of isolation emerges.[54] First, feminists are suspicious of any system that marginalizes women through isolation, impoverishment, or institutionalization. Second, autonomy, which points to independent (and isolating) living, betrays human flourishing in the image of the triune God. Marginalized isolation challenges a widespread social injustice against persons who, presumably, are not socially productive because of a disability as well as the injustice against those who care for them. Pseudo-independence challenges wrongly the justice due to the other (disabled or otherwise) as an integral part of the human community. Marginalized isolation violates the interdependence that defines human beings as human beings.

The contexts of care in the United States reveal both promise and distress. The promise may be found in the hundreds of thousands of secure elders, and the distress may be found in the millions whose long-term dependence becomes catastrophic.[55] Contrary to the suspicions of many, adult children in the United States do not either abandon their parents as an inconvenience or send them off to the nearest (or farthest) nursing home as they become progressively more needful of domestic care. Rather, these aged parents are home, either in their own homes, to which their children frequently visit, or they are moved into the homes of their children. Home becomes the site of increasingly demanding informal care with a concomitantly increasing need for social systems to support the contra-glamorous work of domestic care.[56] On an even darker note, home becomes a place of confinement *for the patient and caregiver alike* and masks the 'house-poor' material crises that sustained care incurs.[57] The circumstances of social constructs on "the family" and the subsequent "hands off" policy of formal healthcare contribute to the proliferation of home care and demand a reevaluation of the (in)justice currently meted to patients and their caregivers. As Martha Holstein argues,

Home care provides a lens through which to view complex relationships between cultural assumptions, public policy, and private lives. These interactions result in practices that raise questions about care, justice, and welfare rights, the relationship of women (and other informal caregivers) to the state, complex meanings of autonomy, especially the conditions of dependency, and the gendered nature of work. Home care illuminates the gender and class injustices that are historically endemic to American social welfare policy.[58]

Home care isolates patients and their caregivers in ways that support the status quo of healthcare in the United States. As long as 'someone' is home to attend to the interdependent relations of the not yet or no longer socially productive, healthcare and social policy in respect of the very young, the disabled, and the frail elderly need not change. The challenges from this sector of the workforce remain silenced by the headline issues heralding autonomy in reproductive, therapeutic, or right-to-die choices. The personal that feminists recognize is political remains behind the closed doors of our own homes. Chronic care and care for people who are disabled remains undervalued labor on one hand and, on the other hand and however still undercompensated, praised as saintly and ideally selfless.[59] As noted earlier, women assume the caregiving responsibilities of domestic maintenance–bathing, clothing, and feeding–in greater numbers than do men.[60] This disproportionate number of women in the domestic (formal or informal) workforce raises concerns over the likelihood that these women are exploited or oppressed by complacence and the expectations that this work becomes them as it does no others.

Justice calls us to attend to those who are marginalized by their need for or their giving of chronic care. That anyone should be marginalized is cause for concern for people who claim personal liberty as a hallmark virtue: the marginalized cannot exercise liberty. But justice demands restitution not of their liberty by itself but of the right-taking of their places with us. The fee-for-service and the US Medicaid/Medicare system has too long sequestered or institutionalized our elders and other chronic infirmed or homebound people with disabilities; a first challenge to US healthcare is to offer adequate compensation to the caregiver for her labor or her time away from the more financially secure public workforce as well as trained respite care for her and her charge.[61] That anyone should be marginalized is cause for concern for people who claim to be created in the relations of imago dei: the marginalized are not, by definition, in real relational union with others, save their own. But justice demands reconciliation of right-relations with others and with God. Current US healthcare practices jeopardize those relations; a second challenge reintegrates caregivers and remembers those who have lost their way back to the social order of their communities.

Finally, if human flourishing is at all a concern of society then the flourishing of all will depend on the flourishing of every member. The content of justice for patients and their caregivers must reflect attention to their basic physical, intellectual, emotional, social and spiritual needs as does the content of justice for those who are neither yet patients nor caregivers. The interdependent nature of human existence as well as the faithful belief in a triune God whose image we confess demands that proportionate needs and services be distributed to those now in need; we fail to flourish and to thrive when even just one of our members, regardless of his disability, fails.

CONCLUDING REMARKS

I have been arguing that human flourishing depends on embracing the radical interdependence of human existence. This interdependence welcomes the relations necessary to sustain life from first to last breath. Those breaths require nurture, the kind of which family members provide to one another and which, once beyond the natal home, a wider community comes to the fore. The community, dependent as it is upon its members, exists because of its members by mutual relations and social organization. I believe that attention to the physical, intellectual, emotional, social and spiritual interdependence characteristic of human existence is thus everyone's responsibility.

My parents belong to a fairly elite company such that many of my concerns of justice to caregivers do not immediately apply to them. I am concerned that my mother has assumed too many of the care responsibilities for my father because of her nursing experience and the inherited cultural expectations of her role as wife. Nevertheless, my parents are financially secure with their pensions, Social Security, and V.A. benefits for additional medical expenses, and the house is paid; they both have higher education experience and Mom holds a BSN degree; they have a strong, willing and able support system of family and friends; they live in an urban county in NJ with a variety of social programs for seniors;[62] and Mom knows how to access these and other services. These factors guarantee (to the extent that such guarantees hold) my parents' security. Unlike many and in spite of AD my parents are flourishing, the responsibilities of their intimate and social communities to them and with them have been thus far fulfilled.

Of course, I am concerned also with the personal changes affecting my father and how these affect my mother and the rest of our family. In many ways my father is a different man than he was before AD began its course. Some argue that AD permits the 'real' person to emerge from the masks and roles assumed to conform to familial and cultural expectations; some find beasts and others find children.[63] In my father's case both findings are evident: at times he is quite sharp, hurtful, and hateful–and in need then of correction; at other times he is openly affectionate, giving, and kind–and in need then of touch. My father is losing himself and it terrifies. 'Who are you?'–your daughter, 'Who am I?'–my father, John's father, Frank's father, Norman's father, you have six grandchildren, your parents were John and Sanidella Iozzio, you are their youngest son but the patriarch of the family clan, your wife is Mary Chidiac, you live at 81 Crosby, you delivered newspapers, sometimes holding three jobs at once to support your family, you . . . , you . . . , you . . . Remember? Re-member.

David Keck has suggested that Alzheimer Disease is a particularly apt metaphor for theological reflection on personhood and purpose, that it is the "Theological Disease."[64] AD disrupts our normally operative denial of death and weakness as integral parts of the human condition as it reminds us of our own finitude and dependence upon others and God; AD tests our obedience to 'honoring our parents' with long-term dementia care; and AD invites us to enter into the mystery of communion with God and with the church to whom we belong. Additionally, AD challenges the cultural paradigm of independence with a theological anthropology of (trinitarian) relationality, while engaging self-care, fidelity, and good humor.

I began these reflections with recent experiences I have had with my Mom and Dad. I am concerned with how my mother will manage the daily routines of care for herself and for my father, whose living is now compromised by AD. The writing on the wall is quite clear: AD is slowly destroying any semblance my father once understood of his life and will be the death of him, that destruction challenges the rest of us to find ways to engage him and keep him secure. If we are to remain faithful to him we must remember for him and sustain the relations that he nurtured. If we are to succeed at this faithfulness we must take care of ourselves and laugh even at the expense of our liberalized autonomy and fleeting independent self-control.

NOTES

1. *The American Heritage dictionary* (1994), s.v., "dignity."

2. I am thinking here of Attention Deficit and Hyperactive Disorders, developmental disabilities, and various degrees of paraplegia.

3. For example, it is just as likely that a husband will assume the responsibilities of care, including bathing, feeding, and toileting, for his wife or a father for his child. See L. E. Herbert et al., "Is the risk of developing Alzheimer's Disease greater for women than for men?" *The American Journal for Epidemiology* 153 (2001) 132-136.

4. Stephen Post argues two essential moral challenges of AD. "First, it requires that we overcome the stigma associated with dementia, principally by being with deeply forgetful persons in attentively caring ways that draw upon their remaining emotional, relational, and creative capacities. Second, it requires that we think carefully about ethical issues arising over the progression of disease and, in particular, that we avoid burdening these persons with invasive medical treatment that, because they lack insight into the purposes of such treatments, constitutes an assault." Stephen G. Post, *The Moral Challenge of Alzheimer's Disease*, 2nd ed. (Baltimore: Johns Hopkins University, 2000) 3.

5. See Albert R. Jonsen and Stephen Toulmin, *The Abuse of Casuistry* (Berkeley: University of California, 1988) and James F. Keenan, SJ, and Thomas A. Shannon, Ed., *The Context of Casuistry* (Washington, DC: Georgetown University, 1995).

6. On these virtues see James F. Keenan, SJ, "Proposing Cardinal Virtues," *Theological Studies* 56 (1995) 709-729. Further, recall that habits or particular ways of acting become virtues only when they are infused with the right reasoning of prudence (see Thomas Aquinas *Summa theologiae* 1.2. 55.4).

7. I will argue that these doctrinal truths lend themselves to an elaboration of the interdependence indicative of the all human relationships.

8. Among other critiques of liberalism, see David Fergusson, *Community, Liberalism and Christian Ethics* (New York: Cambridge University, 1998); Joseph J. Kotva, Jr., *A Christian Case for Virtue Ethics* (Washington, DC: Georgetown University, 1996); Alasdair MacIntyre, *After Virtue*, 2nd ed. (Notre Dame: University of Notre Dame 1984).

9. *The Catechism of the Catholic Church* likewise recognizes this interdependence. "Nothing exists that does not owe its existence to God the Creator" (no. 338) and "Creatures exist only in dependence on each other, to complete each other, in the service of each other" (no. 340). *Catechism of the Catholic Church* (henceforth *CCC*), (New York: Paulist Press, USCC, Inc.–Libreria Editrice Vaticana translation, 1994).

10. Catherine Mowry LaCugna and Michael Downey, "Trinitarian Spirituality" in M. Downey, ed., *The New Dictionary of Catholic Spirituality* (Collegeville: Liturgical, 1993) 980.

11. Consider the dearth of texts or articles attending seriously to what the doctrine of the Trinity may have to say to moralists.

12. See *CCC* no.s 249-256.

13. Aquinas, *Summa theologiae* 1. 29.4c, 36.2c. Further, "The structural comparison between *De Deo uno* and *De Deo trino* [ST 1, 2-26 and 27-43 respectively] indicates that in *De Deo uno* Aquinas worked out that the nature of God is to be To-Be. In *De Deo trino* he shows that the To-Be of God is To-Be-Related." Catherine Mowry LaCugna, *God For Us: The Trinity & Christian Life* (New York: HarperCollins, 1991) 152-153.

14. Aquinas, ST 1. 28.1c, 3c.

15. Aquinas, ST 1. 28.4c.

16. "The Church uses (I) the term "substance" (rendered also at times by "essence" or "nature") to designate the divine being in its unity, (II) the term "person" or "hypostasis" to designate the Father, Son, and Holy Spirit in the real distinction among them, and (III) the term "relation" to designate the fact that their distinction lies in the relationship of each to the others." *CCC* no. 252.

17. Aquinas, ST 1. 29.4c.

18. Aquinas, ST 1. 32.2c.

19. *CCC* no. 238-248. LaCugna also argues that, "The economy is 'proof' that God is not being-by-itself but being-with-us. The sphere of God's being-in-relation is the economy of creation and redemption in which the totality of God's life is given. We have no direct or immediate access to God's being in-itself or by-itself . . . the divine essence is indeed revealed, given, bestowed in Christ, but what is given is not an impersonal nature, an 'in-itself', but the highest, most perfect realization of personhood and communion: being-for-another and from-another, or, love itself." LaCugna, *God For Us* 246.

20. "The God who is thrice personal signifies that the very essence of God is to be in relation, and thus relatedness *rather than the solitary ego* is the heart of all reality" (emphasis mine). Elizabeth A. Johnson, *She Who Is: The Mystery of God in Feminist Theological Discourse* (New York: Crossroad, 1992) 215-216.

21. Not a one of us has achieved what appears and is commonly referred to as independence without having been first dependent (and radically so) on others.

22. "Aquinas crystallizes this development [of relationality] with his definition of persons as "subsistent relations." This means that the persons are persons precisely *as* mutual relations and not as anything else apart from their mutual bonding. Relationality is the principle that at once constitutes each trinitarian person as unique and distinguishes one from another. It is only by their reciprocal and mutually exclusive relationships that the divine persons are really distinct from each other at all. Their uniqueness arises only from their *esse ad*, from their being toward the others in relation." Johnson, *She Who Is* 216.

23. Aquinas, ST 1. 79.2 and 93.5.

24. "Furthermore, this [Trinitarian symbol for God] indicates that the particular kind of relatedness than which nothing greater can be conceived is not one of hierarchy involving domination/subordination, but rather one of genuine mutuality in which there is radical equality while distinctions are respected." Johnson, *She Who Is* 216.

25. Aquinas, ST 1. 76.1c, 5c and 91.3c.

26. Aquinas, ST 1.2. 94.2c.

27. "The trinitarian God, moreover, cannot be spoken about without reference to divine outpouring of compassionate, liberating love in the historical world of beauty, sin, and suffering, thus leading us to envision a God who empowers human praxis in these same directions." Johnson, *She Who Is* 216.

28. Aquinas, ST 1.2. 3.8c and 109.5c.

29. See Stephen J. Duffy, "Friar Thomas D'Aquino: Grace Perfecting Nature" in his *The Dynamics of Grace: Perspectives in Theological Anthropology* (Collegeville: Liturgical, 1993) 149-156.

30. See Martha B. Holstein, "Ethics and Alzheimer's Disease: Widening the Lens," *Journal of Clinical Ethics* 9 (1998) 13-22.

31. See Nancy L. Mace and Peter V. Rabins, *The 36-Hour Day*, rev. ed. (Baltimore: Johns Hopkins University, 2001), "Chapter 2: Getting Medical Help for the Impaired Person;" and *Time*, July 17, 2000: 51-57.

32. 20 million people worldwide, 4 million in the US, are suspected of having AD. *Time*, July 17, 2000: 51.

33. Since writing this article, and subsequent to its review for this journal, my father's diagnosis has been confirmed. AD medications have been withdrawn, leaving him only with a regulating dose of insulin and a drug to control his Parkinson's tremor. Further, with the advance of kidney failure and the decision to not initiate dialysis, my father now receives the additional support of hospice home health care.

34. Aquinas, ST 1.2. 9 and 10. See also James F. Keenan, SJ, *Goodness and Rightness in Thomas Aquinas's Summa Theologiae* (Washington, DC: Georgetown, 1992) especially chapter 3.

35. Consider the questions of competency and/or the determination of personhood based on "intelligence quotients" and the like. See, for example, Allen Buchanan and Dan Brock, "Competence and Incompetence," *Millbank Quarterly* 64 (1986) 67-80 and John D. Arras, "The Severely Demented, Minimally Functional Patient: An Ethical Analysis," *Journal of the American Geriatrics Society* 36 (1988) 938-944 (both reprinted in John D. Arras and Bonnie Steinbock, ed., *Ethical Issues in Modern Medicine* (Mountain View: Mayfield, 1999); and Joseph Fletcher, "Four Indicators of Humanhood–The Enquiry Matters," *The Hastings Center Report* 4 (December 1975) 4-7.

36. "Individuals with dementia have residual strengths. Building on these strengths will improve their functioning and quality of life." Post, *The Moral Challenge of Alzheimer's Disease* 15.

37. See Post, *The Moral Challenge of Alzheimer's Disease*, chapter 3, "Fairhill Guidelines on Ethics and the Care of People with Alzheimer Disease" and chapter 5, "The Humane Goal: Enhancing the Well-being of Persons with Dementia."

38. At this juncture a discussion on suffering and care would be helpful; however, the parameters of this article prevent exploration. Along the lines of thought on interdependence, mortality, and caring see Henri J. M. Nouwen, *Our Greatest Gift: A Meditation on Dying and Caring* (New York: HarperCollins, 1994).

39. This article focuses only on these virtues as they may be sustained and developed by those who are for and about persons with dementia; I do not mean to suggest, however, that persons with dementia cannot sustain or develop virtue.

40. From William Bennett, *The Book of Virtues* (New York: Simon & Schuster, 1993) to Stanley Hauerwas and Charles Pinches, *Christians Among the Virtues* (Notre Dame: University of Notre Dame, 1997), among many others.

41. Although according to a principle-based ethics my father would be deemed incompetent and lacking autonomy, he definitely has considerable control over himself. He remains quite stubborn or quite submissive when he sees it to be to his advantage. Additionally, he inserts himself often into conversations, sometimes appropriately, sometimes inappropriately–or so it seems to us. Nevertheless, these insertions remind us that he is still an important part and an important member of our family.

42. See James F. Keenan, SJ, *Virtues for Ordinary Christians* (Kansas City: Sheed & Ward, 1996), chapter 11, "Self-Esteem."

43. Although for all intents and purposes my father now lacks a distinct sense of self, he is still my father. As such, he is still owed by me the respect due to him as father and by others the respect due to him as a human being. On these same lines, see Stanley Hauerwas, "Must a Patient be a Person to be a Patient? Or, My Uncle Charlie is not

much of a Person but he is still my Uncle Charlie," reprinted in Stephen Lammers and Allen Verhey, ed., *On Moral Medicine*, 2nd ed. (Grand Rapids: Eerdmans, 1998) 387-390.

44. Mary Lucy Chidiac married Francis Anthony Iozzio, May 1, 1949.

45. David Keck devotes much of his text to memory, hope and reconciliation. "[Caregivers] find themselves charged both with remembering another person and with remembering *for* another person. Their daily experience with someone else's diminishing cognitive faculties heightens their sense of trying to remember the patient. However world-historical or simple, the particular experiences shared with a patient become absolutely precious. At the same time, caregivers recognize that they must do the remembering." David Keck, *Forgetting Whose We Are: Alzheimer's Disease and the Love of God* (Nashville: Abingdon, 1996) 207.

46. By abandonment here I do not mean to suggest in any way residence in a specialized facility. The time may come when my mother will no longer be able to care effectively for him and for herself, and that my father will need to be moved from their home to such a facility. I suspect that my mother would visit him everyday.

47. This paraphrase is derived from Aquinas', and Augustine's, definition of virtue; ST 1.2. 55, 4c.

48. Thomas Aquinas, *Commentary on Aristotle's Nicomachean Ethics*, Book Four, Lecture XVI, "Amusement," trans. C.I. Litzinger, OP (Notre Dame: Dumb Ox Books, 1994), no. 851; see also ST 2.2. 168.2c.

49. For an extended discussion on humor, see Robert C. Roberts, "Sense of Humor as a Christian Virtue," *Faith and Philosophy* 7 (1990) 177-192.

50. See Keenan, *Virtues for Ordinary Christians*, chapter 20, "Humor."

51. When Aquinas, commenting on Aristotle, considers friendship in adversity he recognizes that "extraneous pleasure lightens sorrow." Aquinas, *Commentary on Aristotle's Nicomachean Ethics*, Book Nine, Lecture XIII, "Friends Needed in Both Prosperity and Adversity," no. 1931.

52. See also Stephen Sapp, *When Alzheimer's Disease Strikes* (Palm Beach, FL: Desert Ministries, Inc., 1996) 22-24.

53. Disability studies critiques this dualist prejudice against defects of the mind as much as it challenges a dualist rejection of uncontrolled bodies. See Leonard J. Davis, ed., *The Disability Studies Reader* (NY: Routledge, 1997).

54. See Elaine Brody, *Women in the Middle: Their Parent-Care Years* (New York: Springer, 1990); Post, *The Moral Challenge of Alzheimer's Disease*, chapter 2, "The Family Caregiver: Partnership in Hope"; and more recently, Martha Holstein, "Home Care, Women, and Aging: A Case Study of Injustice" in Margaret Urban Walker, ed., *Mother Time: women, aging, and ethics* (Lanham: Rowman & Littlefield, 1999).

55. As Marilyn Martone has recognized, the financial costs of long-term care, whether acute, sub-acute or extended care, require either a declaration of indigence or great personal wealth. See Marilyn Martone, "Making Health Care Decisions without a Prognosis: Life in a Brain Trauma Unit," *The Annual of the Society of Christian Ethics* 20 (2000) 309-327.

56. See Christine Firer Hinze, "Dirt and Economic Inequality: A Christian-Ethical Peek Under the Rug," *The Annual of the Society of Christian Ethics* 21 (2001) 45-62.

57. In her high heels, matching pearl earrings and necklace, June Cleaver most informal caregivers are not; more than likely, they are Cinderellas, with neither prospects of a princely ball to attend nor hope for another's help for any extended period of time.

58. Holstein, "Home Care" 227.

59. . . . and thus suspect from the feminist critique of its control over a woman's place. See Emily Abel, *Who Cares for the Elderly? Public Policy and the Experience of Adult Daughters* (Philadelphia: Temple University 1991), "Representations of Caregiving."

60. Up to three-quarters of formal and informal home caregivers are women. Certainly husbands and sons do contribute to the care of their spouses/parents; however, men are more likely than women to pay a home care worker. Paid in-home service suggests also the long history of economic advantage men have enjoyed *at the expense of their mothers' and wives' at-home or low-income work*. See Holstein, "Home Care" 230-235.

61. As of 2002, the last year for which complete statistics are available, the average hourly wage of home health aides was $6.72; by November 2003, average wage increased to $7.23 (*http://www.bls.gov/oes/current/oes399021.htm#nat*). In particular, note the "Job Outlook" section of the US Department of Labor Bureau of Labor Statistics for home care providers: "Excellent job opportunities are expected for this occupation, as rapid employment growth and high replacement needs produce a large number of job openings. Employment of personal and home care aides is projected to grow much faster than the average for all occupations [in this broad service personnel category] through the year 2012. The number of elderly people, an age group characterized by mounting health problems and requiring some assistance, is projected to rise substantially. In addition to the elderly, however, patients in other age groups will increasingly rely on home care, a trend that reflects several developments, including *efforts to contain costs by moving patients out of hospitals and nursing care facilities as quickly as possible*, the realization that treatment can be more effective in familiar rather than clinical surroundings, and the development and improvement of medical technologies for in-home treatment. In addition to job openings created by the increase in demand for these workers, replacement needs are expected to produce numerous openings. The relatively *low skill requirements, low pay*, and high emotional demands of the work result in high replacement needs. For these same reasons, many people are reluctant to seek jobs in the occupation. Therefore, persons who are interested in and suited for this work–particularly those with experience or training as personal care, home health, or nursing aides–should have excellent job opportunities." United States Department of Labor, Bureau of Labor Statistics, "Personal and Home Care Aides," *http://www.bls.gov/oco/content/ocos173.stm*; accessed January 17, 2005, emphasis added.

62. As of this writing, the availability of many of these services is in jeopardy. State and county support for elders has been reduced drastically. My mother has since secured the services of an elder-care lawyer, who has begun to recommend changes to their joint assets.

63. See Mace and Rabins, *The 36-Hour Day*, chapters 3, 7, and 8: "Characteristic Problems of Dementia," "Problems of Behavior," and "Problems of Mood."

64. Keck, *Forgetting Whose We Are*, "Introduction" and chapter 1, "Deconstruction Incarnate."

RESPONSES TO
"THE WRITING ON THE WALL"

Theological, Personal, Universal: Responses to "The Writing on the Wall"

H. Rutherford Turnbull III, JD

SUMMARY. Rud Turnbull, author of the first essay in this volume, and the parent of an adult son with developmental disabilities, responds to M. J. Iozzio's article reflecting on her mother and father and Alzheimer's disease. Rud notes the theological, personal, and universal virtues of her essay. Alzheimer's disease and other disabling conditions compel people to seek the meaning it has for their lives. Like Dr. Iozzio, Rud Turnbull notes his own appreciation for the role of humor and faith. *[Article copies available for a fee from The Haworth Document Delivery Service: 1-800-HAWORTH. E-mail address: <docdelivery@haworthpress.com> Website: <http://www.HaworthPress.com> © 2005 by The Haworth Press, Inc. All rights reserved.]*

H. Rutherford Turnbull III is Co-Founder and Co-Director, Beach Center on Disability, The University of Kansas, Lawrence, KS 66045.
Printed with permission.

[Haworth co-indexing entry note]: "Theological, Personal, Universal: Responses to 'The Writing on the Wall.' " Turnbull, H. Rutherford. Co-published simultaneously in Journal of Religion, Disability & Health (The Haworth Pastoral Press, an imprint of The Haworth Press, Inc.) Vol. 9, No. 2, 2005, pp. 75-78; and: *End-of-Life Care: Bridging Disability and Aging with Person-Centered Care* (ed: Rev. William C. Gaventa, and David L. Coulter) The Haworth Pastoral Press, an imprint of The Haworth Press, Inc., 2005, pp. 75-78. Single or multiple copies of this article are available for a fee from The Haworth Document Delivery Service [1-800-HAWORTH. 9:00 a.m. - 5:00 p.m. (EST). E-mail address: docdelivery@haworthpress.com].

KEYWORDS. Relationships, family, disability, meaning, humor, faith

The virtues of M. J. Iozzio's "Writing" are tri-partite: theological, personal, and universal. The theological virtue is her argument that relationships, as manifest in the Trinity, are the "stuff" of human existence and of our relationship with God. The personal virtue is her moving description of her family's (especially, her mother's) response to AD in her father. And the universal virtues are her sometimes-stated argument that the challenge of AD is also the challenge of other cognitively limiting disabilities, whether they obtain at birth or thereafter in the life of a family member.

Ms. Iozzio promises to contrast the principles of autonomy with the principles of relationships, but it seems to me that she does not explore the relationship quite enough. True, she must choose her emphasis, but perhaps in other writing she would invite us into her family's life and suggesting answers to such questions that arise from her powerful account in "Writing," as these: What would happen to Mom and Dad, and to the author and other family members, if Mom were to be more autonomous and less caring of Dad? What would happen if we were to ask Dad what he would want of us, especially of Mom (assuming he could tell us in a way that mimics his original competence)? What would his answer be, and how would we honor it (if indeed we would)? I am not as concerned that Ms. Iozzio pays scant attention to the principles of justice and beneficence and non-maleficence as I am that could dig more deeply into the matter of autonomy. I hold that concern principally because she holds strong views about the U.S. health care system, which itself undoubtedly values "autonomy" for both the patient and the physician.

But I quibble, so I return to the virtues of this article. As to the theological: I am not trained in theology; I am hardly even a casual reader in that discipline. I found, however, that Ms. Iozzio's exposition about relationships–the One God in Three–was fascinating. As a raised Episcopalian and current Congregationalist, I find that she, a Roman Catholic, "speaks" to my heritage and offers all Christian (and perhaps other sectarian/faith community members) access to her and to our own thinking about ourselves and our God.

As to the personal, I doubt that any person who maintains the bonds of "original" family after reaching his or her adulthood–that is, any adult who remains in relationships to one's father or mother or both–can escape the dilemma the author describes: how to care for another whose condition dramatically alters the original relationship, and at the same time to recognize and "flourish" in a new relationship. Ms. Iozzio's personalization of this challenge is engaging and dramatic; it brings us into her life and makes us reflect on our own. As parents, we spend years establishing and modifying relationships with our children; but as children, we do not always have the luxury of time to establish new relationships with our dependent parents. If AD or other slow acting debilitative conditions offer us anything positive, it may be the opportunity to enter gradually and carefully, not precipitously and perhaps less than carefully, into new relationships within our families.

Finally, as to the universal, Ms. Iozzio characterizes AD as the "condition" that elicits the theological inquiry and resolution, but she could as well have hypothesized other conditions that do likewise. Some of those conditions are "with us"—us, the family—from birth: the newborn who has innate cognitive or physical limitations/disabilities. Others come to us later and unexpectedly: traumatic brain injury, spinal cord injury, or war-related disability.

All, however, give us—is "give" the word to use here? are "oblige" and "require" more apt?—the challenge and the opportunity to "grow" existentially and theologically. To "grow" may poorly describe what we must do when we confront disability-related revolutions in our lives; perhaps "morph" or "change" is a better way of putting it, for not everyone of us "grows" as a result of being in a crucible.

The question, at least in my life, is not "what is mental retardation" (as it "is" in my son, as it is a defining trait of his), but, rather "what about it"—what is its meaning to him, his family, and others?

Ms. Iozzio invites us, all of us who are affected by the "ab-normal" limitations of a family member, to join with her in asking the "so what" and "why" questions. In accepting her invitation to journey to the existential realm, we come to understand more about ourselves and our relationships with our family and our God, and we find, surprisingly, that "good" can come from "bad" and that humor is an appropriate and even necessary response, together with the others she lists. That single point—that "amusement" exists—warrants a word or two.

In a much-too-serious context—the caring for another and for self—humor can ease the chronicity of care-giving. Perhaps the *Journal of Religion, Disability & Health* would do well to explore, in a series of articles, the role of Acquinas' "amusement" in the caring/health-making process.

Here, let me digress a bit to make the point. From time to time, I have been faced with extraordinary challenges arising from my own or my family-members' ill-health. Especially at those moments, I revert to prayer, sometimes in the sanctuary of simple churches or elaborate cathedrals, sometimes with the aid of the "old" Book of Common Prayer, but usually in silence: at the oddest of moments, the old prayers resurrect themselves in my memory and I offer them up to my God.

As I do, I simultaneously trot out my own abbreviated "12-step" method for sustaining myself. I call it my "Three F" and "Three D" technique for finding some modicum of "salvation," emotionally and spiritually. The three "Fs" are "Faith, Family, and Friends." The three "Ds" are "Doctors (for which you should read 'professional help'), Determination (for which you should read 'courage'), and Dirty Jokes (for which you should read 'dark humor coupled with enlightened amusement and diversion')."

One may find it somewhat sacrilegious to seem to trivialize the challenges of AD or other disabilities and diseases by "F" and "D" mnemonics, but I do not, nor, it seems to me, does Ms. Iozzio.

Faith, family, and friends do sustain us, and we should proclaim that fact, however cute the method of our proclamation. And medicine, courage, and joyous remembrances of the past or projections of the future do, too.

Our Creator has provided us with many graces, many unmerited forms of divine assistance that regenerate us, and we dare not gainsay any one of these.

The Writing on the Wall: Resources for Furthur Reflection

Stanley Hauerwas, PhD

SUMMARY. Stanley Hauerwas notes the strengths of M. J. Iozzio's article and then points to other writers who explore the issues of dependency, relationality, and remembering. *[Article copies available for a fee from The Haworth Document Delivery Service: 1-800-HAWORTH. E-mail address: <docdelivery@haworthpress.com> Website: <http://www.HaworthPress.com> © 2005 by The Haworth Press, Inc. All rights reserved.]*

KEYWORDS. Alzheimer's disease, relationality, dependency, human

I have read this article, and I certainly think it is an essay we should publish. Indeed, I think it's a wonderful essay that begins the kind of discussion surrounding Alzheimer's we do desperately need. It is well written and well argued, and I think could be more or less accepted as is.

I did think the author might want to think about a bit of rearrangement. Starting off with the theological anthropology of relationality doesn't clearly help the author say why she needs to develop that account of relationality. I wonder if she doesn't need to start with some of

Stanley Hauerwas is affiliated with The Divinity School, Box 90967, Duke University, Durham, NC 27708.

[Haworth co-indexing entry note]: "The Writing on the Wall: Resources for Further Reflection." Hauerwas, Stanley. Co-published simultaneously in Journal of Religion, Disability & Health (The Haworth Pastoral Press, an imprint of The Haworth Press, Inc.) Vol. 9, No. 2, 2005, pp. 79-80; and: *End-of-Life Care: Bridging Disability and Aging with Person-Centered Care* (ed: Rev. William C. Gaventa, and David L. Coulter) The Haworth Pastoral Press, an imprint of The Haworth Press, Inc., 2005, pp. 79-80. Single or multiple copies of this article are available for a fee from The Haworth Document Delivery Service [1-800-HAWORTH, 9:00 a.m. - 5:00 p.m. (EST). E-mail address: docdelivery@haworthpress.com].

Available online at http://www.haworthpress.com/web/JRDH
© 2005 by The Haworth Press, Inc. All rights reserved.
doi:10.1300/J095v9n02_07

the stories of the struggle of her father and mother with Alzheimer's disease. That way the readers will be drawn into the subject in a way that they will see the point in the first section once it is appropriately contextualized.

It struck me, by the way, that the author might want to discuss Alasdair MacIntrye's *Dependent Rational Animals* as part of the case she's making. That book clearly establishes how the issue of dependency is at the heart of the human.

I suppose I should also express my worry about whether you really need the doctrine of the Trinity to establish the dependent character as well as the relational character of our lives. G. H. Mead did quite well with an account of relationality of the very nature of the self without any Christian convictions at all. H. Richard Niebuhr, who had a modalist view of the Trinity, also developed a very impressive account of the self's relationality. The author could get some help from Miraslav Volf who argues very much like she does in *In Our Own Likeness*.

I thought the points about remembering are extremely important. I think the author develops that quite wonderfully. But if she wants a source that would help her develop that further, she might look at Joel Shuman's book, *The Body of Compassion*.

This is an outstanding article, and I look forward to seeing it published.

Person-Centered Planning and Communication of End-of-Life Wishes with People Who Have Developmental Disabilities

Leigh Ann Kingsbury, MPA

SUMMARY. Person-centered planning is a common practice in most developmental disability systems. As people with disabilities are living to old age and being supported in the community as they age and die, there is an ever increasing need for advance care planning for people who have developmental and intellectual disabilities; that is, the organizing of advance directives. Since many people already have a person-centered plan, the author suggests that use of a good planning process might be a logical next step for helping people communicate their end-of-life wishes. The author is clear that this is not about active or passive euthanasia, but is about helping people clearly communicate their wishes in the context of increasing age, significant infirmity or terminal illness. *[Article copies available for a fee from The Haworth Document Delivery Service: 1-800-HAWORTH. E-mail address: <docdelivery@haworthpress.com> Website: <http://www.HaworthPress.com> © 2005 by The Haworth Press, Inc. All rights reserved.]*

Leigh Ann Kingsbury is Gerontologist, InLeadS, Wilmington, NC 28405 (E-mail: Kingsburyla@ec.rr.com).

[Haworth co-indexing entry note]: "Person-Centered Planning and Communication of End-of-Life Wishes with People Who Have Developmental Disabilities." Kingsbury, Leigh Ann. Co-published simultaneously in Journal of Religion, Disability & Health (The Haworth Pastoral Press, an imprint of The Haworth Press, Inc.) Vol. 9, No. 2, 2005, pp. 81-90; and: *End-of-Life Care: Bridging Disability and Aging with Person-Centered Care* (ed: Rev. William C. Gaventa, and David L. Coulter) The Haworth Pastoral Press, an imprint of The Haworth Press, Inc., 2005, pp. 81-90. Single or multiple copies of this article are available for a fee from The Haworth Document Delivery Service [1-800-HAWORTH, 9:00 a.m. - 5:00 p.m. (EST). E-mail address: docdelivery@haworthpress.com].

Available online at http://www.haworthpress.com/web/JRDH
© 2005 by The Haworth Press, Inc. All rights reserved.
doi:10.1300/J095v9n02_08

KEYWORDS. Person-centered planning, advance care planning, Essential Lifestyle Planning, PATH

As more and more people with labels of developmental disabilities are welcomed into their communities and are living in communities of their choosing; as more and more people with disabilities are experiencing self-determination (or some attempt from the system to support the principles); and as more and more people with developmental disabilities are living to old age, the need to think about advance care planning, including wishes about extraordinary treatment, advanced directives and health care agents/proxies increases. Disability or no, Americans are not generally well-prepared to address end-of-life issues. It is a subject we avoid until a crisis hits. Nationally, it is estimated that at least 50% of people have not made their wishes known to someone else (personal communication, Ellen Cameron, MSW, Lower Cape Fear Hospice, April 2002). For people with developmental disability labels (such as mental retardation), the assumption is that that figure is even higher. This issue is not just about becoming critically or terminally ill, or having a disability that compromises one's health. This is about being self-determined and planning for one's life . . . *from beginning to end.* Self-determination should not start and stop at some mythical age. It does not stop when one gets old or when one is diagnosed with a potentially terminal illness. Self-determination ought to be about one's entire life.

"Person-centered planning has become the norm" (personal communication, Michael Smull, July, 2001). In many states, person-centered planning is legislated. If done well, we include in individuals' person-centered plans their friends, families, paid and non-paid supporters, their hopes, dreams, fears, clinical concerns, support needs, etc. End-of-life wishes and plans ought to be an integral part of an individual's person-centered plan, too, especially if that person is very ill, aging or old. Having a developmental disability is not a prerequisite either. Good person-centered planning is equally effective with people who have dementia or other acquired disabilities. To be clear, this is not about passive or active euthanasia. This is specifically about helping people communicate their wishes (advance care planning) should they be unable to do so at some point in their lives. Although we spend much of our lives figuring out "how to live," we rarely figure out what we want the end of our life to look like (assuming we have some measure of control over that at all). In the field of developmental disabilities, we have championed person-centered planning as a means for people to convey what is important in their lives and convey the way they choose to live their lives. We know that the core values of person-centered planning include autonomy for the person, attempting to honor his or her wishes while balancing health and safety and supporting interdependence, companionship and relationships. In using person-centered planning to help someone communicate end-of-life wishes, those values do not change.

One of the many questions to be addressed, and certainly not to be answered entirely here, is "how do we remain ethical and mindful as we use person-centered planning to help someone communicate end-of-life wishes, especially someone who is dying?" Botsford and Force (2000) have addressed this question to a certain degree:

> Despite the fact that we each may have unique views about end of life, we need a core set of values to guide our decisions and actions in supporting people with intellectual disabilities . . . (There are) four principles that are applied in bioethical dilemmas . . . (1) respect for the autonomy of the person; (2) do no harm; (3) do what is good and; (4) justice.

As mindful person-centered planners, we should expect to apply those same principles if we were helping someone document and communicate his/her end-of-life wishes and/or if we were helping to support someone who was dying.

Knowing this, and knowing that many people receiving supports and services already have a planning process in place in their lives, it makes sense to use person-centered planning to help people identify their wishes; for example, whom the person would like to have present if they were dying, how the person would like to be made comfortable if he/she requires support to do so, what kinds of treatment/intervention he/she wishes to have or not have, what type of religious or spiritual support he/she wants, etc. For people who do not use words to communicate (people with the label "non-verbal") and for people who use augmented communication devices, writing this information down ahead of time is crucial. Not using words to talk is not the same as not communicating or having nothing to say. Most of us know many people who communicate quite clearly with behavior. Planning ahead and establishing an on-going conversation with the people in the person's life who may be called upon to make an end-of-life decision should the person be unable, is a critical step. It may never be words from which we learn the information needed; but knowing someone well over time, how they communicate with their behavior and having that information up-to-date and written down may be exactly the information that decision makers will need.

It is imperative that the person who is dying has his/her physician as an ally, in addition to other clinicians, family members and friends. Anyone who has had the experience of trying to make end-of-life decisions at the eleventh hour knows that planning ahead of time is a much better alternative. Surrogate decision making may challenging enough without the burden of not knowing someone's clear wishes and having a means to support those wishes. Again, this article is not intended to answer all these questions, but rather open a dialogue for thinking about ways to address them.

Additionally, holding conversations about end-of-life wishes with legal guardians is critical. For the many people who receive supports and services away from their family's or guardian's home, and especially people who have little or no family involvement in their lives, paid direct support professionals are likely to be providing the day-in and day-out support. Those professionals usually care deeply about the individual with disabilities. They may even describe their relationship as "we're like family." They may also have a very clear idea of what they believe the person's wishes would be because they know the person well or because they have actually engaged in that conversation with the person. If, however, the legal guardian's wishes differ from the person's (assuming the person's wishes are known), and if the guardian chooses to act on his/her wishes, direct care staff and others who know and love the person may be deeply saddened, angry and confused over the choices that are made.

Several years ago I had the experience of providing support to a group of direct support professionals when someone they cared deeply for had died. Unbeknownst to them, the guardian made the decision to end nutrition and hydration. At that point, the staff were visiting the man in a nursing home. When they showed up and discovered this situation, they were terrified. Some agreed with the decision; some did not. That was not this issue. They clearly had no decision making authority. Their only role at that point was to visit and provide companionship, but having supported the gentleman for many years, they loved him dearly and they just did not understand. They had no information. It is unfair to the person receiving supports and services and the people who support and love the person to not have end-of-life wishes conversations well before the time comes to act upon those wishes.

Even if everyone intimately involved in the care and support of the person is not on the same page or does not hold the same beliefs, it is helpful for everyone to have a clear understanding of what to expect when the time comes. This is not to imply by engaging in advance care planning that "when the time comes," everything will go smoothly or that it will be "easy." A dear friend died of brain cancer several years ago; it was a slow and devastating process in his and his family's life. When he died, a little more than 3 years after his diagnosis, his wife said "no matter what I thought about 'how ready' we were . . . we were not. I was absolutely not ready to lose my spouse . . . and no amount of planning (which we did a lot of) would have made me any more 'ready.'"

Advanced care planning and communication of end-of-life wishes involves numerous parties: the person, the spouse, the family, the guardian, the provider, caregivers, friends, medical professionals, etc. We need to understand that end-of-life decision-making, like good person-centered planning, is not an *event* but an *on-going process*, and there must be a series of conversations, ultimately leading to decisions, based on the person's, family's, guardian's experiences, values and beliefs. Trying to have these conversations, and make decisions and plans when people are under extreme stress, when they are sad and frightened makes no sense. One of the keys to ensuring that this already-stressful-time is not made even tougher is good, on-going communication. One means of ensuring that communication is to recognize the person's and family's (or guardian's) wishes in the individual's person-centered plan.

One of the cornerstones of person-centered planning is action planning: a way to ensure that the people involved in helping to implement the plan follow through and are communicating with each other. One of the many ways that person-centered planning has always differed from traditional habilitation or treatment planning is that meetings are not just held annually to meet regulatory requirements. By coming together as needed and when it makes sense for the person and his/her family, on-going communication is supported and encouraged and the person's ever-changing life can be supported.

In looking at two of the most tried and true methods of person centered planning, Essential Lifestyle Planning (ELP), and Planning Alternative Tomorrows with Hope (PATH), one can see where each of these processes would be helpful to an aging or dying individual and the people who are supporting him or her. ELP helps people who are planning with and supporting someone to listen, learn, understand and act on what is both important *to* and important *for* the individual with whom planning is being done (Smull, 2001). In the context of planning with someone who is aging and or dying, ELP can help the person and caregivers specifically identify the important rituals, routines, supports, treatments and wishes of the aging or dying person.

In *Twelve Weeks in Spring*, June Callwood (1986) tells the story of Margaret and her "care team," the men and women who circle around Margaret to support her to die at home. Throughout *Twelve Weeks in Spring*, Callwood recounts numerous examples of rituals that bring Margaret comfort and allow for some consistency in her life, as her care team members come and go on a daily basis. There is the way the birds must be fed; the way Margaret's tea must be fixed; the blanket Margaret uses as she curls up on her loveseat in the living room (even though some care team members believe her bed upstairs would be so much more comfortable); the ways Margaret wishes her care team members would keep her kitchen organized (as she did when she was well). Through the implementation of ELP, daily rituals that are vitally important to the person for a sense of routine and comfort, such as special mugs for tea and feeding the birds are not only identified, but are explained and understood as being *important to* the person in his/her daily life. A terminal illness might change the importance of those rituals, but it also may not. Understanding their role in the person's everyday life and how they should be carried out is one important aspect of an ELP.

For a little more than seven years, I had the joy (and adventure) of supporting my grandmother in my home. With support from a wonderful husband and my mother, my grandmother was able to stay home with the support she needed following a severe stroke. For nearly the 80 years prior to her stroke, "Granny" drank Sanka coffee. Following her stroke, her tastes changed and she no longer enjoyed coffee. Short-term memory losses combined with a strong Scottish stubbornness, however, meant that the ritual of coffee after dinner was usually not to be denied. So, for many of the seven years that she lived after the stroke, we fixed a cup of coffee after dinner. Reminding her "but you don't like coffee anymore" was futile. This was not so much about the flavor of coffee as it was a ritual of comfort. It is just what "you did after dinner." Since it always went down the drain, I suppose we were fortunate it was Sanka and not Starbucks brand!

In PATH, one begins the process with the "north star"; or the "where are you going . . . what is your dream?" question. Faye Wetherow, a gifted PATH trainer and facilitator says "when you ask people their dreams, you are walking on sacred ground" (personal communication, Faye Wetherow, May 2000). When people choose to share their dreams with us, they become vulnerable. What if we laugh? What if we disagree? What if we say it is impossible? When someone is aging, slow-ing down, becoming sick more frequently, or when someone is dying, it is easy to become more focused on the clinical aspects of life: medications, pain management, trips to the doctor, therapeutic treatments, etc. This is not to say that those aspects are not important; in fact, it may be impossible to focus on anything else until one's pain is reduced. How often though, do we ask someone who is aging or dying what his/her dreams are? Would we feel uncomfortable asking that question of someone who was dying?

In the context of end-of-life, dreams will likely look very different than they do for someone who, for example, is moving into his/her first apartment or looking to move from sheltered employment to a job in the community. As people age and sometimes slow down, we may forget about the question of dreams. We may wrongly assume that the person is "content" in their daily life and routine; which he/she may be; but maybe not? Does this mean we should not ask then? Why not ask differently? Why not spend some time exploring the person's dreams? There may be dreams for their loved ones (e.g., a dying woman I knew had a dream that her daughter would always "be okay"); there may be dreams of an afterlife or afterworld. There may be dreams of connecting with loved ones who have already died. Facilitating a PATH with someone who is aging or dying may bring comfort, a sense of respect for the person's wishes and concerns, and perhaps even a sense of inclusion or feeling valued; a sense of "even though I am old or critically ill or dying, what's important to me still matters."

Recently I was asked to provide some guidance for staff supporting a young, dying mother with disabilities. The staff was concerned about helping the young woman "accept" the fact that she was dying and address the questions of healthcare power of attorney, extraordinary treatment, interventions, etc. The young mother had only one concern: her daughter. Although the other questions were important and need to be addressed sooner than later, clearly what was most important to the young woman was her concerns about her daughter. Those concerns had to be addressed first, before she was going to entertain any other topic of conversation. Her end-of-life decisions needed to be addressed in the context of her most pressing concern: what was going to happen to her daughter?

By asking someone what his/her dreams are, people who are supporting the person have a mission and a focus. It may even be that using any good person-centered planning process with someone who is aging or dying may also bring comfort to the caregivers; by establishing a clear set of expectations, defined by the person and those who love that person, caregivers may find that they feel more competent and more useful because they know they are doing something that is clearly important to and important for the individual, as defined by that individual. Using PATH, some of those things could be clearly laid out for the caregivers/supporters. Under the category of "first steps," very specific tasks are identified and participants in the PATH can claim responsibility.

Using person-centered planning as the springboard for advance care planning absolutely requires courage and it absolutely requires that one be thoughtful and mindful. The first time I had an end-of-life conversation with a family whose son was dying (and a family I knew well), I was well prepared, had all my ducks in a row and was sure I was ready to go. Upon opening my mouth to begin the conversation, a different scenario emerged. My palms were sweaty, my heart was racing, and one would have thought I had a mouth full of peanut butter and crackers. "Person-centered planning raises, and can productively contain, many difficult ethical issues. . . . Practitioners have an obligation to be thoughtful and courageous about when and how they plan with people" (O'Brien and O'Brien, 2000). Very few issues will raise one's discomfort in the way that discussions around death and dying will. It used to be sex that made us uncomfortable and was a taboo subject, now it is end of life!

In Washington, DC this year, with support from the Quality Trust for People with Disabilities and the District's MR/DDA, we have just begun the *Life Choice Planners* Project *(LCP)*. LCP was conceived because of the need to address the aging and end-of-life issues that are facing a growing number of people with developmental and intellectual disabilities who currently receive services in the District. The project will use the six core skills of person-centered planning and coaching as established by the Essential Lifestyle Planning Learning Community and using those skills as the foundation for planning, will then layer over that foundation information about aging and end-of-life issues. From there, in year one, we will develop a small cadre of planners who will receive hands-on support and mentoring to become skilled coaches around aging and/or end-of-life issues, including such topics as how to balance what is important *to* a person while also ensuring that what is important *for* is addressed; the importance of daily, cultural, spiritual, etc., rituals; how to address issues of grief and bereavement; supporting people who have dementia, etc. Because each end-of-life scenario is unique to the dying person, the coaches' skills will be around good planning and access to resources, not specifics about diseases and terminal illness (though some of that learning will naturally occur). One of the issues that seems to matter a lot to agencies and staff is "what do we do once we know someone is dying?" We hope that through LCP we will develop a network of people who feel somewhat more at ease with this question and have a toolbox of skills and resources to coach the people who are actively supporting the dying individual.

Why should we help people who have developmental disabilities communicate end-of-life wishes? They have a right to be active participants in their healthcare, just as people without disability labels. People with disabilities, their spouses, loved ones, friends, family members, guardians, provider staff, etc., need to know and understand what the options are. Physicians and other medical care providers need to have a greater understanding of the abilities of people with developmental disabilities and their right to be an active part of this planning process. Advance care planning should be a part of everyone's life, whether one has a disability label or not. Without communicating one's wishes, loved ones are left to make decisions of which they are often unsure and which could be in conflict with what the individual would desire. Use of a person-centered planning process should not, and in many places cannot preclude the use of a specific form or process for one's advanced directives and the naming of one's health care agent (durable power of attorney, healthcare proxy, etc.), but a thoughtfully considered person-centered plan can be the foundation for developing more formal directives.

Clearly one of the issues that must be addressed on an individual basis is that of decision making and informed consent. The purpose of this article is not to sort through that specific issue, however it bears mentioning as we learn more about how people with disabilities wish to participate in advance care planning. The Gunderson Lutheran Respecting Choices Program on Advance Care Planning suggests there are four components to capacity.

1. The ability to understand that one has authority–that there is a choice to be made.
2. The ability to understand information–elements of informed consent.
3. The ability to communicate a decision and the rationale for it.
4. The ability to make a decision which is consistent with one's values and goals and which remains consistent over time.

Though not developed specifically for people with developmental or intellectual disabilities, the components may be one reasonable set of standards with which to begin the discussion. Furthermore, there is much additional literature on evaluating the capacity of individuals without mental retardation which has been can be used as a guideline for assessing "capability" for those with intellectual disabilities (personal communication, Barbara Wheeler, 2004). Overlaying that knowledge with the issues of advance care planning is one next logical step in this discussion.

The use of person-centered planning ought to support conversations around what is important to and important for the person; what matters in everyday life; what the person's values are; what their hopes, dreams and fears are; what supports are needed for the person to have a meaningful and quality life on their terms; and how all of those elements can be supported and honored as the person ages, acquires a disability and/or is dying. Self-determination applies to one's whole life—and advance care planning, which can be accomplished as part of trusting and mindful person-centered planning, must be a part of the process.

REFERENCES

Botsford, Anne L. and Force, Lawrence T. (2000). *End-of-Life Care: A Guide to Supporting Older People With Intellectual Disabilities and Their Families*. (2000), Albany: New York, NYSARC, Inc.

Callwood, June. (1986). *Twelve Weeks in Spring*. Toronto: Key Porter Books Limited.

Gundersen Lutheran's Respecting Choices Organization & Community Advance Care Planning Course. Information available at *www.gundluth.org/web/ptcare/eolprograms.nsf*

O'Brien, John and O'Brien, Connie Lyle. (2000). In John O'Brien and Connie Lyle O'Brien (Eds.), *A Little Book About Person Centered Planning* (p. 8). Toronto: Inclusion Press.

Smull, Michael W. (2001). "Seven Questions That Those Who Support People with Disabilities Should Be Able to Answer." Available by request from: Allen, Shea and Associates <*www.allenshea.com*>.

THE LAST PASSAGES PROJECT RESOURCES

End-of-Life Care for People with Developmental Disabilities: Philosophy and Recommendations

For many years, advocates have been demanding equal access, as well as equal rights for people with disabilities. This has resulted in numerous improvements and opportunities for individuals, including the right to plan their own lives, choose their own supports, and live their lives with dignity and respect. The emphasis has been on the similarities, not the differences, with the choices and opportunities afforded other people in our communities. No longer are institutional placements considered an acceptable alternative for individuals with developmental disabilities who need supports. Increasingly, the services are provided under Home and Community Based waivers, which vary in each state, but are all focused on community based services and natural supports. Over the years,

Reprinted with permission from Volunteers of America (http://www.albany.edu/aging/lastpassages/index.htm).

[Haworth co-indexing entry note]: "End-of-Life Care for People with Developmental Disabilities: Philosophy and Recommendations." Co-published simultaneously in Journal of Religion, Disability & Health (The Haworth Pastoral Press, an imprint of The Haworth Press, Inc.) Vol. 9, No. 2, 2005, pp. 91-95; and: End-of-Life Care: Bridging Disability and Aging with Person-Centered Care (ed: Rev William C. Gaventa, and David L. Coulter) The Haworth Pastoral Press, an imprint of The Haworth Press, Inc., 2005, pp. 91-95. Single or multiple copies of this article are available for a fee from The Haworth Document Delivery Service [1-800-HAWORTH, 9:00 a.m. - 5:00 p.m. (EST). E-mail address: docdelivery@haworthpress.com].

Available online at http://www.haworthpress.com/web/JRDH
doi:10.1300/J095v9n02_09

ICF-MR facilities have also downsized with the current trend being small group homes of 4 to 6 people. These trends, along with others such as mainstream education, public policy changes and fair housing enforcement, have begun to ensure that people with developmental disabilities have the same rights to community living and participation. As with society in general, people with developmental disabilities are aging, and facing many of the same choices regarding retirement and living options that are faced by each of us. The life expectancy of an individual with developmental disabilities is within 5 years of a non-disabled person, based on current demographics. We have been discussing this issue for several years; assisting people with retirement and health care needs, and now have begun to discuss end-of-life care planning and options for people with developmental disabilities, that mirror the options available to the general public.

Realistically, we must recognize and strive to overcome the barriers that exist to end-of-life planning for people with developmental disabilities, before moving on to best practices and choices. End-of-life decision making is not a single event that occurs when faced with a critical illness, but, rather, an on-going series of choices, based on life experiences, family and friends support systems, as well as health issues. Our philosophy is that individuals with developmental disabilities should be allowed and encouraged to articulate these choices, throughout the course of their lives, so that their wishes can be respected.

We recognize that individuals with developmental disabilities face some unique barriers to end-of-life choices. First of all, they are often in a dependent condition, where others, including well meaning family members and guardians, are making decisions on behalf of the individual. This brings a whole range of legal and ethical issues to the decisions surrounding end-of-life care, particularly in the legal and health care arenas. Add to this barrier, the confusing maze of regulations that accompany the support system often accessed by people with developmental disabilities, and the problems become even more paramount. Many people with developmental disabilities receive services and supports through the Medicaid system, both for acute care and for on-going services. Each state has developed its own set of rules and regulations regarding person-centered planning and legal guardianship options, in addition to "death reviews" and critical incident reporting processes. While we all recognize the rights of individuals with developmental disabilities to exercise choice regarding end-of-life care, we have often failed to provide individuals and their families with the training and support they need to make these choices. Additionally, we have failed to educate the health care community, at times the general public, regarding the differences in facing a terminal illness and living with a chronic disability. Several advocacy groups are, with good reason, expressing a growing concern with discussions of end-of-life care that preclude the use of life sustaining technology that many individuals with severe disabilities use every day. These often heated discussions regarding "futile care" are becoming more common in health care settings across the country as people struggle to make decisions for others, whose right to choice may not be respected.

Given these issues, it is even more important that we recognize planning for end-of-life care as an on-going activity in a person's life, that begins well in advance of a terminal illness. Educating individuals about death, and the rituals accompanying death may be an appropriate place to begin in the natural process of everyday life. In addition to creating educational opportunities to discuss the cycle of life in all of nature, we must not deprive individuals of the opportunity to participate in the rituals of death, such as attending the funeral of a loved one, or visiting a cemetery where a relative is buried, or planning a part of a memorial service for a beloved friend. Teaching skills associated with comforting, recognizing disenfranchised grief and providing opportunities to discuss choices are also some of the first steps in the planning process. End-of-life care decisions may change with the passage of time, based on an individual's life experience, therefore allowing opportunities to discuss these decisions within the context of natural experiences is the best way to begin planning end-of-life choices.

We believe that the full range of choices available in a community should also be available for people with developmental disabilities. Services such as hospice, home health, family support, health care and spiritual comfort should be available to individuals with developmental disabilities, regardless of where they live. The right to die at home should include supportive living residences and group homes that often provide services to people with developmental disabilities. This means that Medicaid funding must be flexible to support changing needs for a person with a terminal illness, direct support professionals and other staff must receive the training and support they need to provide end-of-life care and state and federal Medicaid regulations must treat death as a natural occurrence, rather than a critical incident. While these issues may seem individually, and collectively, overwhelming, much progress has been made in communities across the country to increase funding flexibility and to support choice in end-of-life treatment. Several states have developed protocols pertaining to their Medicaid regulations that treat anticipated death differently than unanticipated death in regulations and investigations. This separate process relieves care-givers of the trauma of investigation and treats death with the dignity and respect it deserves.

Health care providers must receive education in pain management for people with developmental disabilities, particularly as it pertains to end-of-life care. Family members and staff must communicate with physicians and other health care providers regarding an individual's pain, especially when the person is not able to fully communicate to their health care provider. Hospice providers, while willing to provide services, may need training in the particular needs of a person with developmental disabilities and an understanding of the regulations governing Medicaid services, if the person they are serving is receiving services. Several years ago, CMS wrote a letter of clarification concerning ICF-MR regulations and made it clear that hospice services could be delivered in ICF facilities. Unfortunately, states have not uniformly interpreted this letter and barriers to this service delivery still remain.

Perhaps the biggest barriers to end-of-life care choices for people with developmental disabilities, particularly those with mental retardation, is in the legal arena. Conflicting laws and regulations concerning guardianship, informed consent, DNRs (do not resuscitate orders) and related health care decisions are fraught with barriers for individual choice. Planning for end-of-life care must begin with an understanding of state law and the individual's capacity to give consent. Several projects, conducted by bio-ethicists around the country, are researching ways to support and teach choice. Building on the things we learn in these projects, we recognize that teaching individuals about choosing a health care proxy or making choices about advance directives is a lengthy process that must be carefully explained. With the same attitude of individual choice, guardians must endeavor to reflect the choice(s) of their family member or ward when making end-of-life care decisions. Encouraging guardians to make decisions in advance of a critical incident is paramount to sound decision-making.

Decisions must be made with a pro-disability attitude. We must be clear in our advocacy for individuals with developmental disabilities that each person has the right to life, despite the level of their disability. Every person has the right to choose curative care, even in the face of a dismal prognosis. The right to high-quality palliative care should also be fully extended to individuals with developmental disabilities who choose this end-of-life treatment option. Healthcare providers must recognize and value the difference between disability management and prolonging the end of life. We believe that people with developmental disabilities must have access to the full range of end-of-life care options that we want for all our citizens. Working together, in a pro-disability movement, we can insure that our system of care, including long term and acute care options, fully support an individual's choice.

In summary we offer the following observations and recommendations:

- Discussions regarding end-of-life care should not be a formalized one-time event, but rather part of a natural discussion that takes place over time. Opportunities for learning should be maximized and individuals with developmental disabilities should be allowed to participate in their culture's rituals around death, including funerals, remembrances and other activities that occur during the natural course of one's lifetime.
- Training should be provided for legal guardians who are not family members as well as for family members, who may be asked to make decisions regarding end-of-life care for a person with developmental disabilities. This training should include information about choices available to the general public such as hospice, pain management, and treatment options. Legal needs such as advance directives, guardianship paperwork and related issues should also be discussed..
- Advocating for a full range of end-of-life care choices for people with developmental disabilities, including hospice, pain management, organ donation, the right to have decisions legally recognized, and the option to change their mind regarding their end-of-life care wishes.
- Healthcare providers must respect the rights of the person with developmental disabilities to receive the full range of medical options available. People with developmental disabilities must have their pain recognized and treated.
- The Medicaid system must allow the flexibility for a person to exercise their choices regarding end-of-life care. Funding must support the use of hospice or related services within the person's normal living environment. Confusing, conflicting regulations must be eliminated and natural deaths must be treated with dignity and respect, rather than suspicions and investigation.
- The legal system must recognize the choices of people with developmental disabilities and/or their guardians.

End-of-Life Care for People
with Developmental Disabilities:
Bibliography

This bibliography is divided into five sections: End-of-life care for individuals with developmental disabilities, grief and bereavement, developmental disabilities (aging, healthcare, miscellany), advance planning and healthcare decision making, and end-of-life care–general. Pertinent websites are listed at the end.

END-OF-LIFE CARE FOR INDIVIDUALS
WITH DEVELOPMENTAL DISABILITIES

Barbera, T., Pitch, R., & Howell, M. (1989). *Death and dying: A guide for staff serving adults with mental retardation.* Boston: Exceptional Parent Press.

Blanck, P., Kirschner, K., & Bienen, L. (1997). Socially-assisted dying and people with disabilities: Some emerging legal, medical, and policy implications. *Mental and Physical Disability Law Reporter,* 21: 538-543.

Botsford, A. (2004). The status of end-of-life care in organizations and agencies providing services for older people with a developmental disability. *American Journal of Mental Retardation,* 109/5: 421-428.

Botsford, A. (2000a). Integrating end-of-life care into services for people with an intellectual disability. *Social Work in Health Care,* 31(1): 35-48.

Reprinted with permission from Volunteers of America (http://www.albany.edu/aging/lastpassages/index.htm).

[Haworth co-indexing entry note]: "End-of-Life Care for People with Developmental Disabilities: Bibliography." Co-published simultaneously in Journal of Religion, Disability & Health (The Haworth Pastoral Press, an imprint of The Haworth Press, Inc.) Vol. 9, No. 2, 2005, pp. 97-107; and: *End-of-Life Care: Bridging Disability and Aging with Person-Centered Care* (ed: Rev. William C. Gaventa, and David L. Coulter) The Haworth Pastoral Press, an imprint of The Haworth Press, Inc., 2005, pp. 97-107. Single or multiple copies of this article are available for a fee from The Haworth Document Delivery Service [1-800-HAWORTH, 9:00 a.m. - 5:00 p.m. (EST). E-mail address: docdelivery@haworthpress.com].

Available online at http://www.haworthpress.com/web/JRDH
doi:10.1300/J095v9n02_10

Botsford, A. (2000b). Dealing with the end of life. In M. Janicki and E Ansello, (Eds.), *Community supports for aging adults with lifelong disabilities*, 415-432. Baltimore, MD: Paul H. Brookes.

Botsford, A. (1998). Devalued deaths: Integrating hospice care into services for people with disabilities and their families. (Abstract). *Gerontologist*, 31: 146.

Botsford, A., & Force, L.T. (2000). *End of Life Care: A guide for supporting older people with intellectual disabilities and their families.* Albany, NY: NYSARC.

Botsford, A., & Force, L.T. (2000). Cuidado al final de la vida: Una guia de apoyo para envejecientes con incapacidades intelectuales y sus familias. Albany, NY: NYSARC.

Botsford, A., Force, L., & Janicki, M (1999). Supporting people with intellectual disabilities at the end of life: Evaluation of a teaching model for carers and implications for policy. (Abstract). *Gerontologist*, 39: 186.

Botsford, A., & King, A. (In press). End-of-life care policies for people with an intellectual disability: Issues and strategies. *Journal of Disability Policy Studies*.

Brown, H., Burns, S., & Flynn, M. (2003). 'Please don't let it happen on my shift!' Supporting staff who are caring for people with learning disabilities who are dying. *Learning Disability Review*, 8/2: 32-41.

Chaney, R. H., & Eyman, R. K. (June 2000). Patterns in mortality over 60 years among persons with mental retardation in a residential facility. *Mental Retardation* 38/3: 289-293.

Chochinov, H. M. (2002). Dignity-conserving care–A new model for palliative care: Helping the patient feel valued. *Journal of the American Medical Association*, 287/17: 2253-2260.

Community State Partnerships to Improve End-of-Life Care. (November 2001). Advance care planning–Part 1: Approaches for patients from marginalized groups. *State Initiatives in End-of-Life Care*, 12. Available at: http://www.midbio.org/mbc-publications.htm

Jones, A. (2003). Palliative care and people with learning disabilities. *Learning Disability Practice*, 6/7: 30-37.

Kingsbury, L.A. (November 2004). Person centered planning in the communication of end-of-life wishes with people who have developmental disabilities. *Exceptional Parent* 34/11: 44-46.

Lohiya, G., Tan-Figueroa, L., & Crinella, F. (2003). End-of-life care for a man with developmental disabilities. *Journal of the American Board of Family Practice*, 16/1: 58-62.

Rader, R. (June 2003). Editor's Desk: Last Passages. *Exceptional Parent Magazine*, 33/6: 6.

Stein, G. (2003). Promoting palliative care for people with a disability. Social Work Leadership Development Awards–In the Spotlight. Available at: http://swlda.org

Stein, G., & Esralew, L. (2004). Palliative Care for People with Disabilities. In J. Berzoff & J. Silverman (Eds.), *Living with dying*, 499-507. New York: Columbia University Press.

Sterns, H.L., Kennedy, E.A., Sed, C. (2000). *Person-centered planning for later life: A curriculum on death and dying for adults with mental retardation*. Chicago: RRTC Clearinghouse on Aging and Developmental Disabilities.

Tuffrey-Wijne, I. (1997). Palliative care and learning disabilities: The particular palliative care needs of people with learning disabilities are being overlooked. *Nursing Times*, 93: 50-51.

Tuffrey-Wijne, I. (2003). The palliative care needs of people with intellectual disabilities: A literature review. *Palliative Medicine*, 17: 55-62.

Tuffrey-Wijne, I. (2004). Longer lives mean clients must be eased through longer deaths: 2004-10. *Learning Disability Practice*, 7/8: 7.

GRIEF AND BEREAVEMENT

Carder, M. (1987). Journey into understanding mentally retarded people's experiences around death. *Journal of Pastoral Care*, 41: 18-31.

Deutsch, H. (1985). Grief counseling with the mentally retarded clients. *Psychiatric Aspects of Mental Retardation Review*, 4/5: 17-20.

Emerson, P. (1977). Covert grief reactions in mentally retarded clients. *Mental Retardation*, 15/6: 46-47.

Fauri, D., & Grimes, D. (1994). Bereavement services for families and peers of deceased residents of psychiatric institutions. *Social Work*, 39: 185-190.

Harper, D.C., & Wadsworth, J.S. (1993). Grief in adults with mental retardation: Preliminary findings. *Research in Developmental Disabilities*, 14: 313-330.

Hedger, C., & Smith, M.J.D. (1993). Death education for older adults with developmental disabilities. *Activities, Adaptation & Aging*, 18: 29-36.

Hollins, S. (1995). Managing grief better: People with developmental disabilities. *Habilitative Mental Healthcare Newsletter* 14/3. Available at: http://www.thearc.org/faqs/grief.html

Kauffman, J. (1994). Mourning and mental retardation. *Death Studies*, 18: 257-271.

Kloeppel, D., & Hollins, S. (1989). Double handicap: Mental retardation and death in the family. *Death Studies*, 13: 31-38.

Lavin, C. (1989). Disenfranchised grief and the developmentally disabled. In K. Doka (Ed.). *Disenfranchised grief: Recognizing hidden sorrow*, 229-237. Lexington, MA: Lexington.

Luchterhand, C. (1998). *Mental retardation and grief following a death loss: Information for families and other caregivers*. Arlington, TX: The Arc.

Luchterhand, C., & Murphy, N. (1998). *Helping adults with mental retardation grieve a death loss*. Philadelphia, PA: Taylor & Francis.

Ludlow, B. (1999). Life after loss: Legal, ethical, and practical issues. In S. Herr & G. Weber (Eds.), *Aging, rights, and quality of life: Prospects for older people with developmental disabilities*, 189-221. Baltimore: Paul H. Brookes.

Murray, G.C., McKenzie, K., & Quigley, A. (2000). An examination of the knowledge and understanding of health and social care staff about the grieving process in individuals with a learning disability. *Journal of Learning Disabilities* 4/1: 77-90.

Raji, O., & Hollins, S. (2003). How far are people with learning disabilities involved with funeral rights? *British Journal of Learning Disabilities*, 31: 42-45.

Service, K., Lavoie, D., & Herlihy, J. (1999). Coping with losses, death, and grieving. In M. P. Janicki & A. Dalton (Eds.), *Dementia, aging and intellectual disabilities*, 330-351. Philadelphia, PA: Taylor and Francis.

Stoddard, K.P., Burke, L., & Temple, V. (2002). Outcome evaluation of bereavement groups for adults with intellectual disabilities. *Journal of Applied Research in Intellectual Disabilities*, 15: 28-35.

Summers, S.J., & Witts, P. (2003). Psychological intervention for people with learning disabilities who have experienced bereavement: A case study illustration. *British Journal of Learning Disabilities,* 31: 37-41.

Wadsworth, J., & Harper, D. (1991). Grief and bereavement in mental retardation: A need for a new understanding. *Death Studies,* 15: 281-292.

Yanok, J., & Beifus, J. (1993). Communicating about loss and mourning: Death education for individuals with mental retardation. *Mental Retardation,* 31: 144-147.

DEVELOPMENTAL DISABILITIES– AGING, HEALTHCARE, AND MISCELLANY

Botsford, A., & Rule, D. (2004). Evaluation of a group intervention to assist aging parents with permanency planning for an adult offspring with an intellectual disability. *Social Work,* 49/3: 423-432.

Braddock, D. (2002). *Disability at the dawn of the 21st Century and the state of the states.* Washington, DC: American Association on Mental Retardation.

Braddock, D. (1999). Aging and developmental disabilities: Demographic and policy issues affecting American families. *Mental Retardation,* 37/2: 155-161.

Edgerton, R.B. (1967). *The cloak of competence: Stigma in the lives of the mentally retarded.* Berkeley: University of California Press.

Flower, C.D. (1994). Legal guardianship: The implications for law, procedure, and policy for the lives of persons with developmental disabilities. In M. F. Hayden & B. H. Abery (Eds.), *Challenges for a service system in transition,* 427-447. Baltimore: MD: Paul H. Brookes.

Gritzer, G., & Arluke, A. (1985). *The making of rehabilitation: A political economy of medical specialization, 1890-1980.* Berkeley: University of California Press.

Groce, N.E. (1997). Women with disabilities in the developing world: Arenas for policy revision and programmatic change. *Journal of Disability Policy Studies,* 8: 177-93.

Hanson, K.W., Neuman, P., Dutwin, D., & Kasper, J. (2003). *Understanding the health care needs and experiences of people with disabilities: Findings from a 2003 survey.* Kaiser Family Foundation Report, available at: http://www.kff.org/medicare/121203package.cfm and in a recent online edition of *Health Affairs*, available as *Uncovering the health challenges facing people with disabilities: The role of health insurance*, available at: w3.552v1.pdf

Herr, S., & Weber, G. (Eds.). (1999). *Aging, rights, and quality of life: Prospects for older people with developmental disabilities*, 189-221. Baltimore: Paul H. Brookes.

Janicki, M., & Ansello, E. (Eds.). (2000). *Community supports for aging adults with lifelong disabilities*. Baltimore, MD: Paul H. Brookes.

Janicki, M., & Wisiewski, H. (Eds.). (1985). *Aging and developmental disabilities: Issues and approaches*. Baltimore, MD: Paul H. Brookes.

Kennedy, J. (2002). Disability and aging–beyond the crisis rhetoric: Introduction to the special issue. *Journal on Disability Policy Studies*, 12/4: 226-228.

Luckasson, R., Barthwick-Duffy, W., Coulter, D.L., Craig, E., Reeve, A., Schalock, R.L., Snell, M.E., Speat, S., Spitalnik, D.M., & Tasse, M. (2002). *Mental retardation: Definition, classification, and systems of supports*. Washington, DC: American Association on Mental Retardation.

National Institute on Disability and Rehabilitation Research. (2003). *Changing concepts of health and disability: State of the science conference and policy forum*. Available at: www.ed/gov/offices/OSERS/NIDRR 14-17

Neri, M., & Kroll, T. (2003). Understanding the consequences of access barriers to health care: Experiences of adults with disabilities. *Disability and Rehabilitation*, 25/2: 85-96.

Pearlman, R.A. (August 1996). Challenges facing physicians and healthcare institutions caring for patients with mental incapacity. *Journal of the American Geriatrics Society*, 44/8: 986-7.

Rizzolo, M.C., Hemp, R., Braddock, D., & Pomeranz-Essley, A. (2003). *The State of the States in Developmental Disabilities: 2004*. Washington, DC: American Association on Mental Retardation. Available at: http://www.cu.edu/ColemanInstitute/stateofthestates

Scheer, J., Kroll, T., Neri, M., & Beatty, P. (2003). Access barriers for persons with disabilities: The consumers' perspective. *Journal of Disability Policy Studies*, 13/4: 221-230.

Silverman, W., Zigman, W., Kim, H., Krinsky-McHale, S., & Wisniewski, H. (1998). Aging and dementia among adults with mental retardation and Down syndrome. *Topics in Geriatric Rehabilitation*, 13: 49-64.

Wittenburg, D. (September 2004). A health-conscious safety net? Health problems and program use among low-income adults with disabilities. *New Federalism: National Survey of America's Families* Series B: B-62. Washington, DC: The Urban Institute.

ADVANCE PLANNING
AND HEALTHCARE DECISION MAKING

Cox, R., & Parkman, C. (March/April 2002). The end-of-life movement: Advance care planning. *Continuing Care*, 20-30.

Day, L.J. (April 2000). Decision making by surrogates. *Critical Care Nurse*, 20/2: 107-11.

Friedman, R.I. (1998). Use of advance directives: Facilitating health care decisions by adults with mental retardation and their families. *Mental Retardation*, 36/6: 444-456.

Kapp, M.B. (1990). Evaluating decision making capacity in the elderly: A review of recent literature. *Journal of Elder Abuse & Neglect*, 2/3-4: 15-29.

Kapp, M.B. (1991). Health care decision making by the elderly: I get by with a little help from my family. *Gerontologist*, 31: 619-623.

Keywood, K., Fovargue, S., & Flynn, M. (1999). *Best practice? Health care decision making by, with and for adults with learning disabilities*. Manchester, UK: National Development Team.

McKnight, D.K., & Bellis, M. (1992). Foregoing life-sustaining treatment for adult, developmentally disabled public wards: A proposed statute. *American Journal of Law and Medicine*, 18/3: 203-32.

Midwest Bioethics Center. (Fall 1996). Health care treatment decision-making guidelines for adults with developmental disabilities. *Bioethics Forum*, S/1-8.

Midwest Bioethics Center. (Undated). *Guidelines for the determination of decisional incapacity. Procedures for ethics committees. Self-assessment tool and resource sheet: A guide to assist in case consultation. Case review checklist*. Kansas City, MO: Midwest Bioethics Center.

Robert Wood Johnson Foundation. (2001). *Grant results brief: National leadership summit on self-determination, consumer direction and consumer control among people with disabilities.* Available at: http://www.rwjf.org

Volicer, L., et al. (2002). Advance care planning by proxy for residents of long-terms care facilities who lack decision-making capacity. *Journal of the American Geriatrics Society*, 50/4: 761-7.

END-OF-LIFE CARE–GENERAL

Beltran, J.E. (Fall 1996). Shared decision making: Ethics of caring and best respect. *Bioethics Forum*, 17-25.

Bradley, E., Walker L., Blechner, B., & Wetle, T. (1997). Assessing capacity to participate in discussions of advance directives in nursing homes: Findings from the study of the Patient Self-Determination Act. *Journal of the American Geriatrics Society*, 45: 79-83.

Field, M. J., & Cassel, C. K. (Eds.) (1997). *Approaching death: Improving care at the end of life.* Washington, DC: National Academy Press.

Martin, D., Emmanuel, L., & Singer, P. (2000) Planning for the end of life. *Lancet*, 356: 1672-1686.

WEBSITES

American Association on Mental Retardation (AAMR) promotes progressive policies, sound research, and universal human rights for people with intellectual disabilities, *www.aamr.org*

American Academy of Hospice and Palliative Medicine (AAHPM) is an organization of physicians and other medical professionals dedicated to excellence in and advancement of palliative medicine through prevention and relief of patient and family suffering by providing education and clinical practice standards, fostering research, facilitating personal and professional development, and by public policy advocacy, *www.aahpm.org*

Arc of the United States works to include all children and adults with cognitive, intellectual, and developmental disabilities in every community, *www.thearc.org*

The **Center for Practical Bioethics** is a freestanding practical bioethics center.

Our vision: A society in which the dignity and health of all people is advanced through ethical discourse and action.

Our mission: To raise and respond to ethical issues in health and healthcare.

Our core value: Respect for human dignity. We believe that all persons have intrinsic worth, and we express this belief by promoting both autonomy and social justice in health and healthcare, *www.midbio.org*

Exceptional Parent Magazine provides information, support, ideas, encouragement and outreach for parents and families of children with disabilities, and the professionals who work with them, *www.eparent.com*

Last Passages is a Project of National Significance funded by the Administration on Developmental Disabilities and the Project on Death in America, *www.albany.edu/ssw/research/endoflife.html* and *www.uic.edu/orgs/rrtcamr/endoflife*

National Hospice·and Palliative Care Organization (NHPCO)'s Vision: A world where individuals and families facing serious illness, death, and grief will experience the best that humankind can offer. NHPCO's Mission is to lead and mobilize social change for improved care at the end of life, *www.nhpco.org*

National Institutes of Health State-of-the-Science Conference on Improving End-of-Life Care, December 6-8, 2004, *http://consensus.nih.gov/ta/024/024EndOfLifepostconfINTRO.htm*

Not Dead Yet was founded on April 27, 1996, shortly after Jack Kevorkian was acquitted in the assisted suicides of two women with non-terminal disabilities. In a 1997 Supreme Court rally, the outcry of 500 people with disabilities chanting "Not Dead Yet" was heard around the world. Since then, eleven other national disability rights groups have joined NDY in opposing legalized assisted suicide and euthanasia, chapters have taken action in over 30 states, and helped put Jack Kevorkian behind bars in 1999, *www.notdeadyet.org*

NYSARC, Inc., the largest not-for-profit organization serving individuals with mental retardation and other developmental disabilities and their families. NYSARC has a rich history of providing advocacy and services throughout New York State, *www.nysarc.org*

Quality Mall, a place where you can find lots of free information about person-centered supports for people with developmental disabilities. Each of the "mall stores" has departments you can look through to learn about positive practices that help people with developmental disabilities live, work and participate in our communities and improve the quality of their supports, *www.qualitymall.org*

Rehabilitation Research and Training Center on Aging and Developmental Disabilities, Department of Disability and Human Development, University of Illinois at Chicago. The RRTCADD promotes the successful aging of adults with intellectual (mental retardation) and developmental disabilities (I/DD) in response to physical, cognitive, and environmental changes. Its coordinated research, training, and dissemination activities promote progressive policies and supports to maintain health and function, self-determination, independence, and active engagement in life. The RRTCADD is a national resource for researchers, people with intellectual and developmental disabilities, their families, service providers, policy makers, advocacy groups, students, and the general community. The RRTCADD is committed to Participatory Action Research. Its active consumer and family advisors and its national advisory board of major disability, aging, and advocacy organizations help insure that the RRTCADD's research is relevant and is responsive to culturally diverse populations, *www.uic.edu/orgs/rrtcamr*

The **State of the States in Developmental Disabilities Project**, University of Colorado, established in 1982 to investigate the determinants of public spending for mental retardation/developmental disabilities (MR/DD) services in the United States, the project maintains a 26-year longitudinal record of revenue, spending, and programmatic trends in the 50 states, the District of Columbia, and the United States as a whole. Analysis of the rich detail of the data base reveals the impact over time of federal and state fiscal policy, and illustrates important service delivery trends in the states in community living, public and private residential institutions, family support, supported employment, supported living, Medicaid Waivers, demographics, and related areas. These financial and programmatic trends are presented in *The State of the States in Developmental Disabilities: 2004,* by Mary C. Rizzolo, Richard Hemp, David Braddock, and Amy Pomeranz-Essley, available at *www.cu.edu/ColemanInstitute/stateofthestates*

SPIRITUAL ENCOUNTERS

Our Last Months with Amber: An Email Reflection

David Wetherow

SUMMARY. An email response by David Wetherow to a question on a community inclusion listserv regarding care for a person whose condition had been defined as 'terminal.' The letter describes the way in which the family provided direction in the final months and days of care provided to their daughter, Amber, by both Faye and David Wetherow and the health care professionals with whom they worked. *[Article copies available for a fee from The Haworth Document Delivery Service: 1-800-HAWORTH. E-mail address: <docdelivery@haworthpress.com> Website: <http://www. HaworthPress.com> © 2005 by The Haworth Press, Inc. All rights reserved.]*

KEYWORDS. End-of-life care, decision making, rights, relationships

---

David Wetherow is affiliated with Communityworks, Canada (E-mail: david@ Communityworks.info) (Website: http://www.communityworks.info).

[Haworth co-indexing entry note]: "Our Last Months with Amber: An Email Reflection." Wetherow, David. Co-published simultaneously in Journal of Religion, Disability & Health (The Haworth Pastoral Press, an imprint of The Haworth Press, Inc.) Vol. 9, No. 2, 2005, pp. 109-111; and: *End-of-Life Care: Bridging Disability and Aging with Person-Centered Care* (ed: Rev. William C. Gaventa, and David L. Coulter) The Haworth Pastoral Press, an imprint of The Haworth Press, Inc., 2005, pp. 109-111. Single or multiple copies of this article are available for a fee from The Haworth Document Delivery Service [1-800-HAWORTH, 9:00 a.m. - 5:00 p.m. (EST). E-mail address: docdelivery@haworthpress.com].

Through our last months in intensive care with Amber, we repeatedly faced the question about whether or not to take the next step in treatment or whether to take the next step in trying to preserve her life in the moments when her life was directly threatened.

As we worked through this question with physicians and nurses—sometimes literally from one hospital shift to another—we were able to become somewhat more articulate about what we were trying to get across (Steve Drake and other allies were very helpful with this). Our instruction to 'save' her life expanded to a request to 'preserve, protect and defend her life,' and we developed additional ways of articulating what we were thinking.

We repeatedly asked people to think in terms of what they would do if Amber were a 23-year-old woman who did not have a disability. Near the end, after a harrowing night when Amber had literally been pulled back from the brink of death, we asked people to act in terms of the deep impulse that led them to save her life in that terrible circumstance.

Ultimately, we asked people to 'do what was possible' in whatever circumstance was arising. "Do what you can do to preserve her life. We understand that there may be a circumstance in which there is nothing that can be done—when we've reached the hard limits of anatomy and physics. But we only find that limit by doing what can be done."

We also requested that in dire circumstances, she would be given sufficient medication to make it possible for her to be free of pain and free of terror.

When we were having these discussions we were faced with people who were directly and forcefully challenging us: "Why are you doing this? Are you just trying to hold on to her for one more hour, or one more day, and tormenting her in the process?" Again and again we carefully tried to help people understand that we were keeping a life-long promise to her and that we were operating in terms of deep principle, and not out of emotion.

The night after that last discussion, we got a 2:00 a.m. phone call.

"She's in serious trouble. We're doing what we can. But we think we may not be able to keep ahead of this one."

By the time we got to the hospital 35 minutes later, the nurse in charge of the ICU met us in the hallway and said, "I'm so sorry. We did everything we could, but we couldn't save her. I need to tell you that we made sure that she wasn't in pain and wasn't in terror."

They kept their promises, and acted with honour, and we bless them for that.

As you journey with your loved one, the way I would translate this position in practical terms would be the following:

- Continue nourishment and hydration [this was the immediate question that had been posted on the listserv]
- Continue support for respiration and heartbeat
- Treat infections
- Provide truly adequate pain control
- Do what can be done, including resuscitation in the event that respiration and heartbeat cease
- Recognize that there will be things that 'might' be done that will not do anything to preserve, protect or defend a person's life, and use principled judgment at the moment to not take those steps
- But don't 'write the person off' (which in my view includes DNR orders) in advance
- In my opinion these steps are humane, loving, principled, and would be fully in accordance with good palliative care.

Former Columnist's Final Words Inspire

Susan Harrison Wolffis

SUMMARY. Susan Wolffis, a columnist for The Muskegon Chronicle, writes about the last days of Paul Novoselick, another columnist who died of multiple sclerosis. *[Article copies available for a fee from The Haworth Document Delivery Service: 1-800-HAWORTH. E-mail address: <docdelivery@haworthpress.com> Website: <http://www.HaworthPress.com> © 2005 by The Haworth Press, Inc. All rights reserved.]*

KEYWORDS. Multiple sclerosis, death, hospice, relationships

TUESDAY, FEBRUARY 01, 2004

For a year, he has bared his soul.

He has talked about living with multiple sclerosis, a devastating neurological disorder that has ruled his days and nights and reined him in even more than he anticipated the past 12 months.

Susan Harrison Wolffis is Columnist, The Muskegon Chronicle, P.O. Box 59, Muskegon MI 49443.

(Editor's Note: This column was sent to us by Richard Rienstra, a friend of Paul Novoselick, the columnist about whom the following column is written. Richard notes: "Paul had quite a sense of humor. Before the funeral service began a screen came down and Paul was recorded in a video with the message: 'This is Paul Novoselick and I approve this message.' " We are grateful to Richard Rienstra for bringing this to our attention, and to Gunnar Carlson, Editor of the Muskegon Chronicle, and Susan Harrison Wolffis, for their permission to reprint this article.)

[Haworth co-indexing entry note]: "Former Columnist's Final Words Inspire." Wolffis, Susan Harrison. Co-published simultaneously in Journal of Religion, Disability & Health (The Haworth Pastoral Press, an imprint of The Haworth Press, Inc.) Vol. 9, No. 2, 2005, pp. 113-117; and: *End-of-Life Care: Bridging Disability and Aging with Person-Centered Care* (ed: Rev. William C. Gaventa, and David L. Coulter) The Haworth Pastoral Press, an imprint of The Haworth Press, Inc., 2005, pp. 113-117. Single or multiple copies of this article are available for a fee from The Haworth Document Delivery Service [1-800-HAWORTH, 9:00 a.m. - 5:00 p.m. (EST). E-mail address: docdelivery@haworthpress.com].

Available online at http://www.haworthpress.com/web/JRDH
doi:10.1300/J095v9n02_12

He has tackled tough subjects: aging, loneliness, the prospect of death.

He has reveled in life's triumphs: providing for his family; doting on his only daughter; making his wife laugh when by all rights, she could have wrung her hands and cried; calling his friends together one last time; teaching a new puppy to jump onto his hospital bed for an afternoon nap.

He has faced people with whom he's had disagreements and apologized; and he's sought reconciliations with others with whom he had mutual misunderstandings.

He's cried when he had to; thumbed his nose at life's trivialities when he wanted to.

And through it all–this roller coaster of emotions and events–he's had a chance few others have.

Paul Novoselick has seen; he's been told; he's been reassured that he made a difference in this community and beyond.

"I know I'm still connected to the outside," he said one day early in January, "because people tell me."

For 16 years, Paul wrote a column in The Muskegon Chronicle, informing readers about the rights and the challenges of the disabled. In his writing, he was activist, advocate, mentor.

Often, he used his own disability to tell the story for those who had no public voice.

A year ago, when he knew his days were numbered, when he was told he was in the end stages of his time on Earth, he did what he'd been doing for much of his career.

Paul Novoselick laid his life open in the pages of the newspaper.

For years, he dedicated his journalistic career to demystifying the plight of the disabled.

In February 2004, he took on one last assignment.

He told a story everyone will one day face–one of death, dying and living until the end with as much joy as one human being could possibly summon from within.

Last Wednesday afternoon, after a couple days of feeling achy and even more fatigued than usual, Paul Novoselick slipped into an unresponsive state.

He could not talk or move. His breathing was labored. He could no longer swallow.

He was at home as he had requested, tended by his wife, Cyndy, who has been his caregiver for 20 years, and Hospice of Muskegon-Oceana, which came to his aid a year ago.

Paul was kept comfortable, but by his expressed and explicit wishes, nothing heroic was done to reverse his medical condition.

Hospice workers told his family it could be a matter of hours, days or maybe weeks before death claimed him. Early Monday afternoon, Paul died at home, a few friends and Cyndy at his side.

Since last week, Paul's family, friends and Lola, the dog the Novoselicks adopted in December, have kept faithful vigil at his bedside.

"It's hard for people to see someone they love in the end stages of life; I know that," he said in an interview on Jan. 12, preparing for today's installment of "Turning the Corner."

"I've seen a lot of people take a deep breath and swallow hard before they come through my door," he said, "and I think some people stayed away because they just didn't know what to say or do once they got here."

The original topic for this month's column was about visiting people who are terminally ill: what to say, how to handle the emotions, what it means to the patient to have someone visit.

"I'm still the same person; honest," he said. "I still laugh. I still like to know what's going on with people . . . if I could go to them, I would, but since I can't . . . they have to come to me."

For 20 years, Paul lived and worked with multiple sclerosis, a neurological disorder that gradually robbed him of clear eyesight and speech, his ability to walk, grip a pencil or operate a computer keyboard.

Not everyone with MS is affected the same way; not everyone's disease takes the same progression.

"Compared to other people, I've had it easy," he said more than once.

No one anticipated that he would take such a dramatic turn for the worse last week.

He went in for his regular dose of chemotherapy Jan. 21, a regimen he followed every few months, taking a drug that, in layman's terms, shrunk the MS plaque in his brain. He was always nauseated, always exhausted, always complained of aches and pains after chemo, but give him a week or so, and he usually bounced back.

Best of all, the chemo seemed to give him a few weeks of energy. Ten days ago, immediately after he had chemo, Paul asked his wife to take him to the Hospice office to say hello to the nurses. Then he wanted a Fricano's pizza.

The next day he jokingly told friends he didn't think the chemo "took"because of the grease from the pizza.

Nonetheless, he asked them to give him a couple days to sleep it off, then they could come over.

On Tuesday afternoon, without warning, he started the long decline into what medical personnel call "an unresponsive state."

By Wednesday, he retreated to a place of transition. From that moment on, the people who love him watched and waited and told their favorite "Novo" stories, while Lola the dog brought him her toys and dropped them on his bed, nudging his hand with her nose. No one knew whether to laugh or cry.

And so they did both.

"Do you tell people you love them?" Paul asked early in January.

He'd had a conversation the day before with a Hospice chaplain about expressing love, and it weighed heavy on his mind.

"I guess I'm like my dad," he said. "It's just not something I say."

It seems the chaplain recommended that he start.

"What do you think?" he asked.

In the beginning, which was just about a year ago, friends took chocolate shakes to the house when they went to visit because they knew he liked them, and besides, it was less awkward to come bearing milkshakes than to tell a co-worker how much he was loved.

Sometimes he had four or five shakes lined up in the freezer at a time. It wasn't until he'd been home from the hospital a couple months he finally told friends chocolate and dairy products upset his digestive system, and he couldn't drink shakes anymore.

"Do you think people will get the wrong idea if I said that . . . if I said I loved them?" he asked.

Someone taped a photograph taken at Christmas of his wife, Cyndy, and his daughter, Alissa, to the television set by his bed. A co-worker and her granddaughter posed with him for the camera, and that picture went up, too. And finally, just a couple weeks ago, someone added a photo of his mother, Julia Novoselick, to his gallery.

"I love you," he started saying to the people in his circle.

Last Wednesday, they were his last distinguishable words. Only Cyndy was with him at the time.

A year ago, Paul made his wife promise he'd never go back to the hospital.

He'd had several brushes with death. In March 2003, he was hospitalized for three weeks with a severe MS "episode," as he described them.

His family was called to his side one night to say their final goodbyes.

But almost miraculously, he rallied with the help of steroids and other medical protocol. In January 2004, he was hospitalized for a week with much the same scenario.

But he said "never again."

Before he left the hospital on Jan. 27, 2004, and went home as a Hospice patient, Paul made his family promise there'd be no medical intervention; and no steroids would be administered. He couldn't bear the steroids' side effects: horrifying hallucinations.

He went home, aware of the realities of his no-intervention decision, but there was no changing his mind. He was at peace with what was to come.

"I never used to pray as a kid," he said as recent as two weeks ago.

Over the last couple months, he talked more about his faith than he ever had. He talked at length about his parents and his blue-collar upbringing and the solid foundation they gave him growing up in Cloverville.

"I went through the motions," he said, "but lately. . . . "

He motioned toward a box tucked on a shelf beneath the television at the side of his bed and asked for help opening it.

"They're my grandmother's rosary beads," he said.

He reached for them and held them close, counting out the number of "Hail Marys" he was supposed to be saying, his hands hardly working.

"I feel like it means something, like there's communication there," he said. "I add my own prayers, of course."

He fingered the beads, lost in thought for a moment, silent.

"I pray for everyone I love," he said.

Index

BOOK ORDER FORM!

Order a copy of this book with this form or online at:
http://www.haworthpress.com/store/product.asp?sku=5712

End-of-Life Care
Bridging Disability and Aging with Person-Centered Care

____ in softbound at $19.95 ISBN-13: 978-0-7890-3073-3 / ISBN-10: 0-7890-3073-X.
____ in hardbound at $34.95 ISBN-13: 978-0-7890-3072-6 / ISBN-10: 0-7890-3072-1.

COST OF BOOKS _____

POSTAGE & HANDLING _____
US: $4.00 for first book & $1.50
for each additional book
Outside US: $5.00 for first book
& $2.00 for each additional book.

SUBTOTAL _____

In Canada: add 7% GST. _____

STATE TAX _____
CA, IL, IN, MN, NJ, NY, OH, PA & SD residents
please add appropriate local sales tax.

FINAL TOTAL _____

If paying in Canadian funds, convert
using the current exchange rate,
UNESCO coupons welcome.

❑BILL ME LATER:
Bill-me option is good on US/Canada/
Mexico orders only; not good to jobbers,
wholesalers, or subscription agencies.

❑ Signature _____

❑ Payment Enclosed: $ _____

❑ PLEASE CHARGE TO MY CREDIT CARD:
❑ Visa ❑ MasterCard ❑ AmEx ❑ Discover
❑ Diner's Club ❑ Eurocard ❑ JCB

Account #_____

Exp Date _____

Signature _____
(Prices in US dollars and subject to change without notice.)

PLEASE PRINT ALL INFORMATION OR ATTACH YOUR BUSINESS CARD

Name		
Address		
City	State/Province	Zip/Postal Code
Country		
Tel	Fax	
E-Mail		

May we use your e-mail address for confirmations and other types of information? ❑Yes ❑No We appreciate receiving
your e-mail address. Haworth would like to e-mail special discount offers to you, as a preferred customer.
We will never share, rent, or exchange your e-mail address. We regard such actions as an invasion of your privacy.

Order from your **local bookstore** or directly from
The Haworth Press, Inc. 10 Alice Street, Binghamton, New York 13904-1580 • USA
Call our toll-free number (1-800-429-6784) / Outside US/Canada: (607) 722-5857
Fax: 1-800-895-0582 / Outside US/Canada: (607) 771-0012
E-mail your order to us: orders@haworthpress.com

For orders outside US and Canada, you may wish to order through your local
sales representative, distributor, or bookseller.
For information, see http://haworthpress.com/distributors

(Discounts are available for individual orders in US and Canada only, not booksellers/distributors.)

The Haworth Press Inc.

Please photocopy this form for your personal use.
www.HaworthPress.com

BOF05